The NICU Mama Survival Guide:

Post-Partum Healing From Your Baby's Bedside

Dr. Heather Evans, DPT

Pelvic floor physical therapist & NICU mama veteran

The NICU Mama Survival Guide

The information in this book is not intended or implied to be a substitute for professional medical advice, diagnosis, or treatment. If you have a medical concern, you should consult with your healthcare provider.

Printed in the United States of America

ISBN: 9798463974365

Prologue

Welcome, mamas.

First of all, congratulations. Congratulations if your baby was born five days ago and is in the NICU now, and congratulations if your NICU baby is now twenty-five. Each NICU journey is unique, and you should be proud of yourself for wading through these waters, even if you weren't really given a choice. NICU mamas are part of a sisterhood, and I believe this extends as well to fathers, aunts, grandmothers, friends, and any other loved one who is close to a child who passes through intensive care. The NICU will change you – it's impossible to take your baby home after a NICU stay and remain the same person you were before. You learn about yourself, your strength, and your resilience during what may be the most terrifying time of your life.

I am a NICU mama myself. My twins were born at 24 weeks, 1 day gestation, and we spent four months in the NICU. I am also a pelvic health physical therapist. This means that I am a physical therapist who specializes in many areas of women's health with much of my day spent treating pregnant and post-partum mothers. So that being said, I knew exactly how to care of myself during my post-partum journey.

I didn't do it. At all.

When thrown into the NICU, I completely disregarded myself, the fact that I had just had a major abdominal surgery, and my entire post-partum recovery. I didn't address my c-section scar until much later, I didn't care about my pelvic floor (remember – full-time pelvic health physical therapist), and I can't remember thinking once that I should focus on myself post-partum. My babies were on ventilators, feeding tubes, and had brain bleeds; I didn't have the space in my brain or the energy in my body to focus on anything other than them. So, while this may sound like what a parent should do, I realize now that there is absolutely no reason to martyr yourself. In fact, I wonder how much better I could have handled the NICU and all of its turbulence if I had put more thought and time into my own recovery. I also realize that by taking care of myself, I would have in no way lost any time with my children while they were in the NICU. It has now been eight years since my NICU experience. That's eight additional years of working with post-partum women, many of whom have experienced their own NICU journeys. Eight years that have given me distance from the trauma I experienced so I can now look back, think everything through, and give advice that I wish I had been given when my world turned upside down.

Having a baby in neonatal intensive care (NICU) is something that can take the breath straight from your lungs, change all your plans, and leave you grasping for control of anything in your life. The plan to bring your baby home two days after birth in that adorable little outfit may be gone. Your baby shower may be canceled or indefinitely postponed. The vaginal birth you imagined may have turned into an emergency c-section. Your sister who was planning to travel to help you after the delivery is several states away and can't take off work this early. Maybe, if you are like I was, you have not even had a chance to tour the hospital.

I was in shock. Not to mention that I was recovering from an emergency c-section with all kinds of drugs coursing throughout my body. My babies were a floor above me fighting for their lives while I could hardly keep my eyes open and had no idea what day it was. It was day 1 in what would become a four-month journey during which time I completely disregarded my own health and recovery. So, I am here today to make sure that YOU do not do the same thing.

Whether this book finds you at the start of your NICU journey, mid-way through, or years later, I hope this information can help you turn inward a bit and focus on what an amazing thing your body did. I want you to love on that little baby as much as you can, but I also want you to love yourself and give yourself the time and energy that you deserve. You have likely heard the age-old reference of putting the oxygen mask on yourself before you help anyone else. We get it in theory, but no one is less likely to do this than a mother whose baby is in the NICU. I'm here to help guide you through so that both your baby AND you can come out on the other side of this, ready to move on strong and healthy when the NICU chapter closes.

It doesn't matter if your baby was in the NICU for three days, three months, or a year. Every baby, and therefore every mother, has their own story, and we all deserve a proper recovery, both physically and mentally, so that we can meet NICU challenges with as much strength as possible.

Big hugs, NICU mamas. I have been there, and I am here for you.

Table of Contents

How to use this book

Everyone's journey is unique so I wrote this book with the idea that some readers may read from the beginning to the end while others may choose to skip around, focusing on the areas that seem most relevant to them. Because of this, please bear with the fact that there may be some slight repetition because certain information is extremely important for different conditions, and I want to make sure nothing is missed. If you have time, I do recommend reading through each chapter because often, women do not realize that something they have noticed about their body is actually related to pregnancy/birth and can be resolved. I have included some questions to ask yourself at the end of each chapter to further guide you wherever you are on your NICU journey.

I also highly recommend finding a pelvic floor physical therapist if your symptoms continue (see Resources section to help find a PT). Please follow-up with your physician regarding any and all symptoms. Please also seek help from a physician, social worker, or counselor if you need further help with mental health issues that are so prevalent when working through the trauma of the NICU.

This book is intended for education purposes and is in no way intended to substitute for medical advice. Please see your physician to address your specific concerns.

I wish you all the best as you begin your healing journey.

Love from one NICU mama to another,

Heather

Our Story

After four years of infertility, four rounds of IVF, and finally, the use of donor eggs, I was finally pregnant with twins – a little boy and a little girl. There had been no real pregnancy complications, and after I had reached twenty weeks gestation, I began to feel great with more energy and less nausea. I also began to let myself think (just a little bit) that this might really happen. I went in for a doctor's appointment at twenty-one weeks, and a transvaginal ultrasound showed shortening of my cervix. This means that basically, instead of dilating from the bottom near my due date, my cervix was dilating from the top at less than six months gestation. I was put on bedrest at home, rechecked, and when things worsened, I was admitted into the hospital at 22 weeks, 5 days. I was given steroid injections to speed up the babies' lung development, another medication to try to stop the labor, and was constantly monitored because apparently, even though I couldn't feel them at that point, I was having contractions.

I stayed on hospital bedrest, but ten days later, labor picked up again and could not be stopped. I was rushed into the operating room and underwent an emergency c-section. My twins, Hannah and Gavin, were born at 24 weeks, 1 day gestation at one and a half pounds each. They were both immediately intubated, Gavin was given chest compressions, and they were rushed upstairs to neonatal intensive care, where they would stay for the next 122 days. They were born so prematurely that their eyes were still fused shut. They were on ventilators for seven weeks followed by further oxygen support for six months. They both had intraventricular hemorrhages (bleeding in their brains from the high levels of oxygen they needed), and Gavin's was the worst level at a grade 4. Gavin received nine blood transfusions, and Hannah received seven. They had more imaging in their first week after birth than most children will have in their entire lives. Gavin had heart vessel surgery at 3 weeks while still weighing only one pound. There were constant alarms, and my husband and I would dash from room to room with the doctors and nurses whenever one of the babies decided to crash. The twins would not be able to breast feed for months, but we were told breast milk was especially important for preemies (micropreemies, to be exact) so I was trying to exclusively pump behind the curtain of the NICU room while my body struggled to understand what it was supposed to be doing sixteen weeks before it was ready.

I ignored my c-section scar. I think I showered once in a while, and I probably ate something. I'm pretty sure I drank water to help with the breast feeding, but I couldn't drink it in the babies' rooms so it was only when I would go home or quickly run to the parent lounge. I never focused on my breathing, but I would guess that I was using shallow, chest breaths. I slept between calls from the NICU at night, and I never thought once about my pelvic floor or recovering from my pregnancy and surgery. Despite my physical therapy background, I didn't care. I never thought about how at one point, the babies would come home and I would need to know how to properly lift them. I just wanted them to live.

The twins came home after four months. They were finally released from their oxygen at six months. At some point, I probably began to breathe again, but I didn't address my muscles or my c-section scar for years even though – remember – I am a PELVIC HEALTH PT. I knew what to do, I just didn't do it, because it didn't rank high on my priority list, and I associated all of it with the trauma of our time in the NICU. Looking back now, I realize that focusing on my recovery would have in no way taken any time, energy, or love away from my children. I hope to use this book to help other NICU mamas, wherever they are in their journey, to care for themselves in the way they deserve.

To read our full NICU story, check out my book, **Learning to Breathe** (see Resources).

Chapter 1:

From a Bun in the Oven to a Baby in the NICU

You grew a human. You freaking grew a human! It doesn't matter if you delivered early or had complications, you are amazing, and you should be proud of your body. So many things happen when you become pregnant, many of which we are blissfully unaware. There are hormonal changes that relax our ligaments in order to prepare for childbirth. Blood volume increases. Center of gravity shifts. Sleep, appetite, bowel movements, urination – everything changes. Some of our NICU mamas carry to nearly 40 weeks and others carry a little over half that long, but either way, there is a moment when you are pregnant and then suddenly...you're not.

If you are reading this and you are post-partum (remember, if your baby was born two days ago, you are post-partum AND if your baby was born five years ago, you are post-partum – there is no time limit!), it helps to understand some of the changes that your body underwent during pregnancy. First, let's start with the hormone relaxin because, while it is helpful for delivery, it can wreak havoc on your system during pregnancy and afterward. Relaxin is a hormone that is produced during pregnancy (beginning in the first trimester and continuing for at least three months after you deliver or stop breast feeding/pumping). Its primary purpose is to increase the laxity (looseness) of your ligaments so that your pelvis can better allow for vaginal delivery. The problem with this hormone is that it isn't produced just right before delivery, it courses throughout your body for most of your pregnancy (and even if your pregnancy was shortened due to preterm delivery, it still has plenty of time to have effects on your pregnant and post-partum body). Sometimes in the clinic, patients will see me during pregnancy with complaints of hip pain, back pain, or pelvic pain. Other women will be fine during pregnancy however once they begin to return to moving around post-partum, they start to notice aches or, even worse, sharp pains. All of this can stem (in part) from relaxin.

So, as I mentioned, this hormone relaxin causes looser ligaments which can lead to more movement at certain joints, including joints that are normally very stable. This commonly affects the SI (sacroiliac) joints which are located on either side of your upper buttocks where your low back meets the arches of your hips. Because of the ligament laxity, your hips may be in a position where one side is a little higher than the other or there is a rotation to one direction. Often, these changes are very small and you might not be able to notice them yourself however a trained physical therapist can check for these alignment issues and help you to correct them. Similarly, many women have pain in their pubic symphysis during pregnancy which is where the pubic bones come together in the front above the vulvar region. This joint almost never causes pain any time other than pregnancy/post-partum (excluding the occasional severe gymnastics straddle injury – *ouch*), and it is because the extra laxity in the ligaments during pregnancy allows this normally very stable joint to have a little movement. By a little movement, I mean a very tiny amount – we're talking millimeters – but it's enough to cause debilitating pain. Some women notice their pubic symphysis pain resolves immediately after delivery however for many women who have this pain during pregnancy, it does not. Lastly, because of the increased joint mobility and decreased stiffness of the ligaments, you can also develop muscle tension. Why? Our bodies crave stability as we move throughout our daily activities. If we are unstable due to pregnancy hormones, our muscles (commonly ones in the back of the hips and inner thighs) jump in – "Hey, we'll help out!" They are trying to help you stabilize however often this tightness can lead to additional pain and even nerve dysfunction. If the tightness in the back of the hips restricts the sciatic nerve, it can lead to pain, numbness, and weakness down one or both legs which is another common complaint heard during pregnancy and post-partum.

Pregnant women often present with what a physical therapist might call an anterior pelvic tilt, but in easier terms, this is the posture one often imagines when they think of pregnancy – a woman whose pelvis is tilted forward with a large sway in her low back. As the baby grows, if women are not actively aware of correcting their posture, they often allow their pelvises to tip more forward than they need to (making it nearly impossible for the abdominal muscles to do their job), also leading to that big low back sway which can lead to further muscle imbalances and achiness. Oppositely, other women present with a posterior pelvic tilt, pushing their hips forward and clenching their glutes.

Now, at this point, you may be thinking, "that would have been good to know during my pregnancy, but now I'm 8 weeks post-partum so what good is this?" Well, don't tune out yet! One thing I see almost daily in the clinic is post-partum mamas who ended up in one of these postures during their pregnancy, and despite having given birth, their posture remains the same post-partum. Also, if you are breast feeding, there is still relaxin in your system so this continues to affect your joints and muscles. By no means is that EVER a reason to consider stopping breast feeding, but instead, learn what you can do to counteract these effects so that you can continue to provide for your little one while feeling much better yourself.

Okay, so what can you do?

1) **Standing posture check:** Dress in something somewhat fitted such as a tank top or a fitted shirt and stand sideways facing a large mirror (you can also prop up a phone and take a full-body selfie if you do not have access to a large mirror). Take a look at your posture. Are your hips and pelvis in line with each other? Are you one of the many women who stand with a forward tilted pelvis and a large sway in your low back? Or, are you like others who stand with their hips pushed forward and their butts clenched? Now see if you can adjust your hips so that your ribs and pelvis are in line. Notice how you can better activate your abdominals. Now that you know what to do in front of the mirror, try it while standing next to your little one's isolette. I notice that for myself and many of my patients, my posture worsens when I am fatigued (physically or mentally). Nothing is more exhausting that the NICU so if you are doing your best to correct your posture, and you notice your body

continues to find its way back to the "not ideal" position, don't beat yourself up about it. Just keep working on it, and you will see improvement in time.

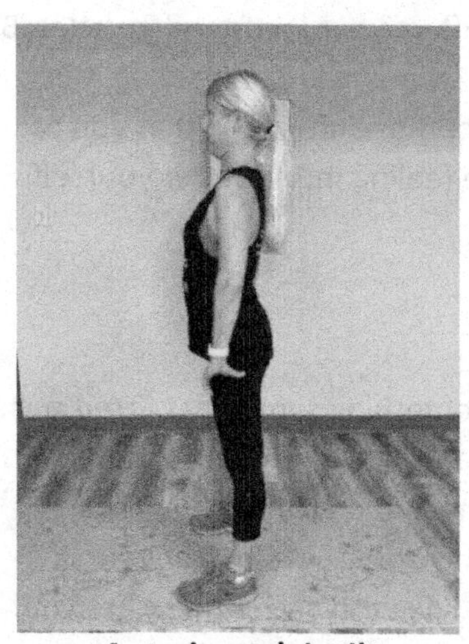

Anterior pelvic tilt

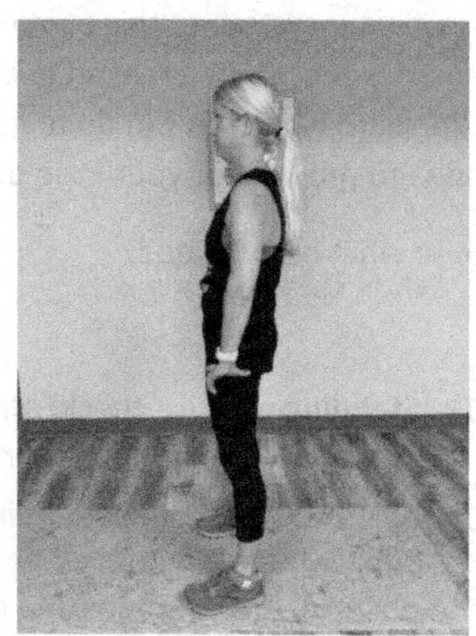

Posterior pelvic tilt

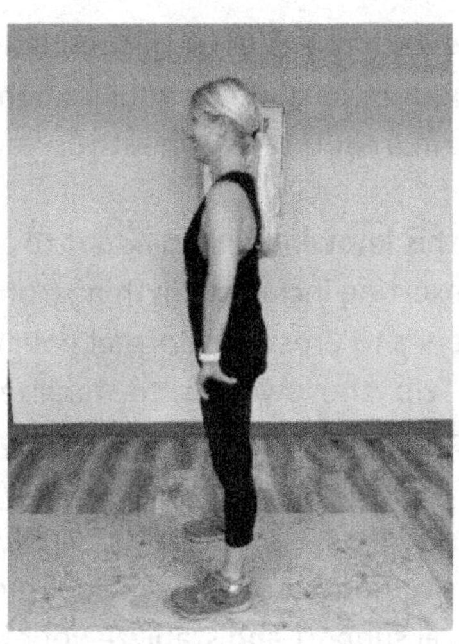

Ribs and pelvis in line – this is the goal!

2) **Zip-it-up exercise:** Now, let's work on activating those abdominal muscles. Many of us are more dominant in our middle and upper abs, but what we want to focus on are our *lower* abdominals. These are our most important stabilizers, and if you contract your upper abs and not your lower ones, it can actually push down on your pelvic floor and pelvic organs. To learn to engage the lower abs, I love the zip-it-up technique. Often, when first learning, this exercise is most easily completed on your hands and knees or laying on your back with your knees bent. That being said, you can certainly work on it while sitting in a chair in the NICU. Imagine you have a vertical zipper that goes from your pubic bone to your belly button. Inhale using your diaphragm by breathing in through your nose and letting your belly expand out (more on this in Chapter 4). Exhale through your mouth and gently "zip" up your lower abdominals from your pubic bone up to your belly button. This is a gentle activation, not a full-on contraction. Hold this for 5 seconds, and then relax. Focus on your lower abs, trying to keep your upper abs at rest. Repeat 10

times, twice each day. If you are completing this exercise sitting in the NICU, be sure to sit up on your sit bones instead of slouching - it can be hard in a NICU recliner, but you can do it!

3) **Now, take this knowledge and add it to any exertion you do in daily life:** (exertion includes anything from turning over in bed to lifting groceries to CrossFit). Correct your posture. Inhale first, then exhale and "zip" the lower abs to stabilize your back and hips. Continue to blow out and stabilize while you perform the movement, such as turning over or lifting. The exhalation will get rid of the air pressure in your body that could push either down on your pelvic floor or out on a weak abdomen. The lower abdominal activation will support and stabilize your body while you complete these movements. When my patients first try this, they are shocked how much better it feels. Get the hang of it in the NICU because someday, when your baby comes home, this is the technique you use to lift your baby and later, your toddler!

4) **Loosen up tight muscles!** Like I mentioned earlier, two culprit areas of muscle tension tend to be the back of the hips and the inner thighs. For the back of your hips, stand with your back to a wall and place a lacrosse ball (available online or at sporting goods stores) between your bottom muscles and the wall. Bend your knees and gently massage the ball all around the back of your hips. Any time you feel tenderness, this indicates a tight area and you want to focus on trying to massage it to get it to relax. Remember, though, keep it to your tolerance. For the inner thighs, sit down and use a rolling pin to massage up and down the inner thighs. If you are pregnant or newly post-partum, I encourage you to go from right above the knee up toward your hip and then, instead of rolling back down, pick up the rolling pin and place it back closer to your knee before rolling it up again. This helps reduce any pregnancy or post-partum swelling.

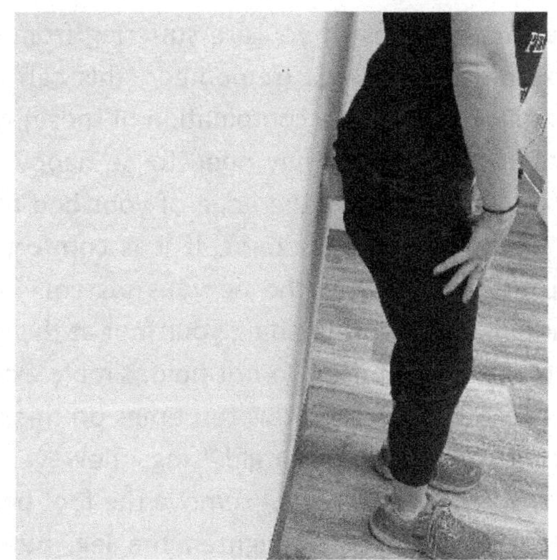

Ball massage to the back of the hip muscles

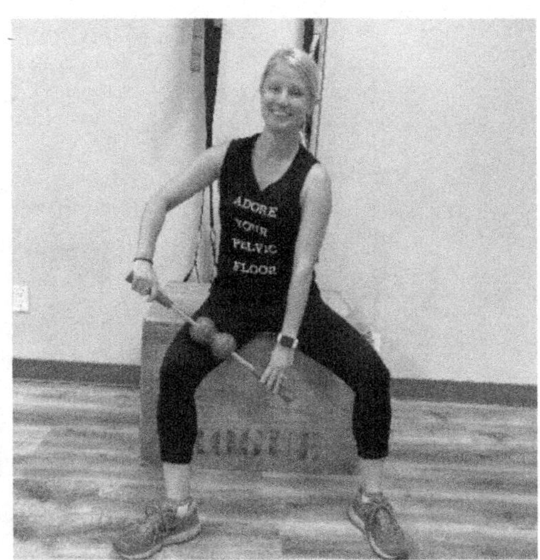

Rolling pin massage to the inner thighs

5) **Move those nerves!** If you are suffering from symptoms traveling down one or both legs (remember, this can be pain, numbness, tingling, weakness, or a combination of these), you want to provide the nerves with what they need to be happy – movement, blood flow, and space. Sit on the edge of your bed or NICU recliner with your hands behind your back. If it is comfortable, go ahead and slump – this lengthens the nervous system. Extend your right leg out until it is straight, bending your foot at the end by bringing your toes toward your nose. Do not hold; simply extend it, then bring it right back down. Repeat this ten times on this side. You may feel a slight muscle stretch or a mild "zing," however you should not feel pain. If you notice pain, first remove the foot bend at the top. If you still feel pain, do not straighten the leg, but instead begin with simply bending and relaxing the ankle ten times each. All of these movements will mobilize (move) the nerves. Repeat on the opposite side ten times.

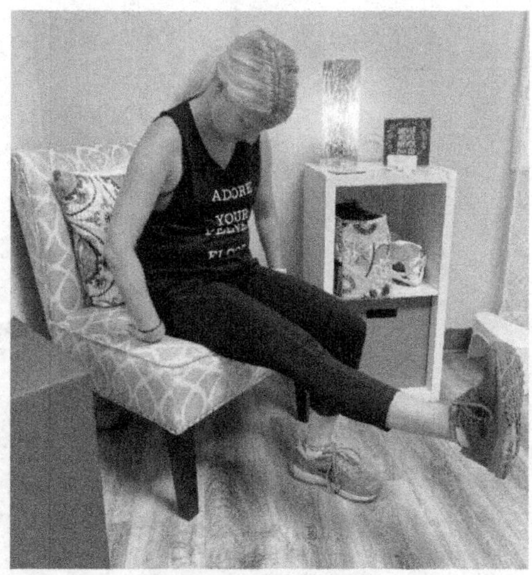

Seated nerve glides

If you are pregnant or post-partum and having back, hip, or pubic symphysis pain, you may also check out the Resources section for recommended support garments, such as SI belts, belly supports, and pregnancy/post-partum leggings. As always, if you continue to have pain, please consult your physician or a post-partum physical therapist.

Questions

1. What was your pregnancy experience like?

2. What was your favorite part of your pregnancy?

3. What was the hardest part of your pregnancy?

4. If you could give advice to someone who is newly pregnant about pregnancy itself, what would it be?

5. Was there anything about pregnancy that you did not expect?

Chapter 2:
"Just Try to Relax:" Bedrest

Bedrest in theory: You get to lounge in your pajamas in your fluffy, king-sized bed while your significant other brings you bowls of ice cream as you watch season after season of Grey's Anatomy.

Bedrest in reality: Your entire world has just been flipped upside down, and you've been forced to sharply reassess your entire plan. First of all, something has concerned your doctor which has led to the bedrest in the first place. So – anxiety up. If you are like me, you may have already decided that you will work up until at least 38 weeks before beginning your 12 weeks of maternity leave. Sudden bedrest - pivot. Maybe you have a toddler at home and well, we all know how easy it is to care for a toddler from the couch since they always listen to every given instruction, right? Piece of cake. Or, in some cases, you are now on bedrest in the hospital. You are now living, without any warning, in a sterile environment where you can no longer take showers and you have to pee in a bedside commode (if you're lucky). You get three hospital meals a day and your husband, if he's able to stay, is stuck sleeping in a plastic recliner while still trying to go to work each day.

And, oh by the way? You have no idea how long this will last, but if you're lucky, it's a really long time.

With my twins, I began with about five days of bedrest at home. I set up camp on our couch. My husband was completely jealous that I got to be off work and relax while I, at the same time, was spending all my time googling "incompetent cervix" which was my official diagnosis (don't even get me started on that term). We all know we shouldn't search the Internet, the doctors tell us not to search the Internet, but when you're stuck on the couch and have been given a scary diagnosis that can affect your unborn child...most of us search the Internet. If you can avoid doing this, it's definitely best, but if you can't, please take nothing at face value and use it only as a resource to help you find specific questions to ask your medical team. Remember, many of the people posting on the Internet may not have accurate information, and often it's the "worst-case scenarios" that you see because the "best-care scenarios" are out living their lives. For good quality Internet resources, please see the Resources section.

Anyway, between googling things I shouldn't have been googling and trying to figure out how many things I could save off Pinterest to make all of my spare time useful, I quickly learned I had a hard time turning off my whirring brain and just relaxing. I expect many readers may be past their bedrest, however for those of you who may be on bedrest right now, I highly recommend getting the book "Pregnancy Brain" by Parijat Deshpande. This is a beautiful book for high-risk pregnancy mamas that can give you a lot of support in working through this time.

I was on bedrest at home for five days followed by an additional ten days in the hospital antepartum unit. When they last weighed me a day or two before the twins were born, I had lost three pounds despite eating everything I could from the cafeteria. I was trying to hydrate well so I figured that most of the weight I lost was from muscle mass in just that short number of days. An inpatient physical therapist came to my room and showed me some exercises that were technically allowed, but I had two babies barely wanting to stay inside of me and I was terrified, so I did a few of the arm exercises and that was it. I was living in fear that if I lifted my hips off the bed in the wrong way, it would send me into labor so the only lower body movement I allowed myself was to the commode and back.

Some NICU mamas have short bedrests, some have none at all, and some have lengthy rest periods. I remember when I was first admitted to the hospital, the nurses told me they wanted me to stay on antepartum as long as possible. They even told me one woman was on antepartum so long she hand-sewed curtains for the room. While I did everything in my power to follow her lead, I managed ten days on hospital bedrest before the twins came. No matter how long you are resting, you lose strength and you need to slowly and healthily build it back up so that you can care for yourself and your little one.

For more details on recovering from birth, please see the chapters "Vaginal Delivery Mamas" and "C-section Mamas." Please know, however, that if you have been on bedrest, especially if it has been for a lengthy amount of time, that it is *very* normal to feel extremely fatigued as you begin to move back into your daily activities. Your stamina will be reduced, and you should never feel like you should be able to "bounce back" quickly from this time. I suggest beginning with short walks. This can begin in the hospital such as around your little one's NICU isolette to start, possibly leading to walks to and from the NICU (although this is highly variable by hospital, how far you have to walk, if you had a c-section, etc. – never feel bad if you are using a wheelchair to and from the NICU as every situation and building are unique). When you are released home, even if it is without your baby, complete comfortable walks within your home. You may find you need frequent rest breaks in the beginning or that you become out of breath doing tasks you find surprising, such as climbing a few stairs. Listen to your body and rest when you need to; I have had patients who had a large number of stairs with a landing in the middle and they temporarily placed a chair on the landing so that they could rest prior to climbing the second set of stairs. Do not push your body to try to immediately return to all daily tasks.

I feel that with myself, as a NICU mama, all of my attention was shifted to my little ones and I almost "forgot," if you will, that I had just had fifteen days of bedrest followed by a major abdominal surgery.

I promise you. Tending to yourself during this time will *not* take anything away from your baby or your care for him or her. If anything, caring for yourself during this time will give you more strength (physically and mentally) to fight the tough NICU fight each day. You *can* care for your baby while also caring for your recovering self at the same time *without sacrificing anything else.*

I also think that with myself, I struggled with guilt for having my twins so early. This is something I have worked on for many years, and I think it is a common theme I hear among NICU mamas (and by all means, please, please seek out a counselor or social worker if you are feeling this way). Because of the guilt I struggled with at the time, I think I subconsciously felt that I did not deserve to focus on recovery from my pregnancy, bedrest, and delivery. I had not carried my twins full-term. I had only been pregnant for six months. Had I been pregnant long enough to even need to recover? Could I even consider myself "post-partum?"

Mamas, eight years later, I can now give you a resounding "YES," you had a real pregnancy, you are post-partum, and you need to recover just as much as the woman in the next hospital room that delivered at 40 weeks. Please use what you can from this book, see a physical therapist if you need to, and if you are struggling as I was, find a counselor or social worker to begin working through any guilt that is impeding your healing.

Sending love.

Questions

1. Were you on bedrest at home or in the hospital (or both)?

2. If you are a recent NICU mama, how has your body felt as you have returned to daily tasks?

3. If your NICU stay was in the past, what can you remember about how your body felt after delivery?

4. How do (or did) you feel about your body and your recovery?

Chapter 3:
Adore Your Pelvic Floor

You may have heard about the pelvic floor in the media or while browsing pregnancy and post-partum websites. However, when my twins were fighting for their lives in the NICU, I didn't care one bit about my pelvic floor and remember, *I'm a pelvic health physical therapist.* Bear with me here, though, because I'm confident now that if women understand what the pelvic floor is and how important it is, they will be more willing to address it especially when I remind you...this can all be done in the NICU, right next to your baby. No time has to be spent away from your little one; it will simply help you improve any problems you might be experiencing while taking nothing at all away from your time as a mother.

The pelvic floor is actually a group of fourteen different muscles that begin around your pubic bone in the front, travel underneath your pelvic organs in three layers like a hammock, and attach around your tailbone in the back. They maintain bowel and bladder continence (keep you from peeing your pants when you sneeze), support your pelvic organs, are involved in sexual functions such as orgasm, and are part of your core stability. We are never taught in health class about this muscle group and how important it is. When I was in physical therapy school, we actually studied the hip and low back and then *skipped over the entire pelvic floor*, moving on to the legs. Don't even get me started. My point, though, is that we don't really think much about this area until something goes wrong.

Now, think about pregnancy. Whether you gained 15 or 75 pounds, that is a significant amount of increased pressure on these pelvic floor muscles. Then, both vaginal delivery and c-section can cause further damage to these muscles (see Chapters 5 and 6). In my opinion, every post-partum mother should be prescribed pelvic floor physical therapy for an evaluation and treatment as needed. In France, all post-partum mothers are automatically given 10-20 pelvic floor physical therapy visits following their delivery. In my clinic, we try to reach as many mothers as we can during pregnancy in order to emphasize how essential it is that the pelvic floor is checked (usually around 6 weeks post-partum or afterward) to address any muscle tension or weakness.

Some of my patients schedule an appointment because they are having symptoms such as painful sex or urinary leakage after a delivery. Often, however, when we dive into their history, the patient may mention things that were present prior to pregnancy like difficulty using tampons, trouble starting a urine stream, or constipation. Some of these patients have a history of pelvic floor dysfunction and then pregnancy and delivery exacerbate the issues until there is more of a problem. Other women have no dysfunction prior to pregnancy, but have trouble afterward. Some women have no dysfunction at all, but I highly recommend all post-partum women (remember, you are still post-partum if your baby is 25!) look through the following chapters to see if they find themselves in any of the descriptions. I can't tell you how many patients I've had come in and say, "well, I had a baby ten years ago so I just thought it was normal to pee whenever I laugh." NO! "I've stopped having sex with my husband because it hurts since I've had my baby." Again – NO! These are all dysfunctions of the pelvic floor, and they can be treated and resolved.

Many women have heard of Kegel exercises, especially in relation to pregnancy and post-partum. If you have not heard of these, they are pelvic floor muscle contractions. I strongly suggest, however, that you do not automatically begin these exercises simply because you are post-partum. While these muscles may be weak and need strengthening, they can also be too tense and in these situations, contraction exercises could make things worse. Imagine a time when someone has massaged the muscles between your neck and shoulder. Tight, right? Maybe some trigger points, often referred to as "muscle knots?" Definitely, I get them all the time. This is how I describe pelvic floor muscle tension to my patients. Just like you can have tension in these neck and shoulder muscles, you can also have tension in your pelvic floor. If the muscles are too tight, adding squeezes to this area might only make the tension worse. The best thing to do is to be evaluated by a trained pelvic floor physical therapist in your area if you are having any pelvic floor symptoms such as urinary leakage, pressure in the pelvic region, or pain with sex. If that's not an option, please read through the rest of the chapters and see where you see yourself falling. If you are someone who has both symptoms of tension (for example, pain with sex) as well as weakness (pelvic organ prolapse or incontinence), always address the tension first and then when that improves, move on to the weakness.

That sounds like a lot, but this can all be done right by your little one's isolette! If it sounds confusing, I promise it will become much clearer as you read each chapter. My second promise is that every single recommendation can be completed without taking any time away from your top priority, your baby.

Questions

1. Have you ever heard of your pelvic floor?

2. If you have, what have you heard?

Chapter 4:
Every Breath You Take

We take about 22,000 breaths each day. If your baby is in the NICU, sometimes your baby's breathing is all you can think about. Babies are hooked up to ventilators, CPAP masks, and nasal cannulas. Babies that do not need oxygen support are still closely monitored, and any dip in oxygen saturation causes concern. Alarms ring throughout the unit, slower and lower pitched for slight oxygen desaturation and higher pitched, frantic alarms if oxygen rates fall further. For the smallest premature babies, they may just simply forget to breathe, and a nurse or parent has to gently shake them or rub their foot to remind them to do this basic life function. What we take for granted each day is a full-time job for premature babies and those with other medical conditions. Anyone who has ever heard the hiss of a ventilator can close their eyes and feel the rhythmic pulse.

What people don't realize is how important breathing is for the rest of us (well, beyond the obvious part). I'm referring to how it can help us naturally move the pelvic floor, regulate pain, decrease stress, and improve sleep and immunity, just to name a few.

Okay, let's start with a test. This can be done on a couch on bedrest prior to delivery, in a hospital bed, sitting in a plastic chair next to an isolette in the NICU, or in your house with your older children running around begging for snacks. This test can be for the current NICU mama or for the NICU mama veteran. There are several ways you can do this, so just pick whatever is most doable for you in the moment.

I want you to watch yourself breathe. Don't change anything – don't try to do things "better" because then you will lose the benefit of this exercise. You can stand in front of a mirror. If you're sitting by an isolette, see if you can catch your reflection in one of the areas of glass or plastic (since, as we all know, there are a LOT of them). If you have a partner with you, give them the directions to watch you. If you are allowed to have your phone in the NICU (even if it's in a plastic bag), turn it to selfie mode and hit video. If you aren't allowed to, take a quick break to visit the restroom or the parent lounge where phones are allowed. If you are like me and have elementary-age kids who think they are budding YouTube stars, give them your phone to video – trust me, they'll think it's awesome. Somehow, I want you to see how your body looks when you breathe. Again, don't change anything you would normally do. Breathe in and out a few times. Take note of how you feel. Are your breaths slow or fast? Where do you notice expansion? Chest? Neck? Belly? Do you breathe through your nose or mouth or both? Do you feel restriction anywhere? Think about how you might feel during a time of stress, and imagine how this might be different.

Now, stop and review your video or think about what you saw if you were watching in real time. Continue to read about how we can adjust our breathing for the best benefit and then analyze again to see where you might make a positive change.

Let me explain what I see in our physical therapy clinic day in and day out. Hang in there, and then I'll explain why it matters and how we can make improvements. From years of sitting in school, offices, and cars, people often begin to breathe with their chests and what we call accessory muscles ("helper" muscles, such as the neck muscles). When you watch your video, did you see a big expansion of your chest? If so, this is you (and most everyone, so don't feel bad). If you are under stress (hello, NICU), this becomes even more pronounced and your breaths become shallow and more rapid. While this is fine for short periods of time, it does not do your body any favors to stay this way for a prolonged period. Looking back, I'm pretty sure I breathed this way throughout our entire four-month NICU stay and the first year of my twins' life.

So. What do we do instead and why?

Diaphragmatic breathing exercise

Your diaphragm is a dome-shaped muscle at the base of your ribs. It is essential for proper breathing, pelvic floor movement, and core stability.

To recruit this muscle, place one hand on your chest and one hand on your abdomen. You can do this laying down or, again, sitting in the plastic recliner next to your baby's isolette. Inhale slowly through your nose for two seconds and focus on expanding your belly and ribs so that you are breathing with your diaphragm as opposed to your chest and accessory muscles. You should feel the lower hand move, but the top hand on your chest should remain fairly still. Your ribs should also move out and up. Then, exhale through your mouth slowly for four seconds. You should feel the belly hand move back and the ribs come back down and in. Some patients prefer to place a hand beneath each side of the rib cage to feel the expansion, and that is fine, too. Continue this breathing for ten breaths and then re-evaluate how you feel.

I'll explain why this is important for all new mamas, and then we'll look at NICU mamas specifically.

When I see post-partum moms in the clinic, this is one of the very first things we address. Your diaphragm sits right below your rib cage, and with pregnancy, it can become "squashed." Add that to the fact that you likely were already breathing with your chest prior to pregnancy, and this means most new mamas come in breathing with their chests. A bit of anatomy info: if you think of your abdomen and pelvis like a canister, the diaphragm is the lid and your pelvic floor is the bottom. These two regions are supposed to move together like a piston, meaning if you breathe in properly, your diaphragm moves down and so does your pelvic floor. This is SUPER important, especially coming from a pelvic floor physical therapy perspective. After delivery (vaginally or c-section), you need this lengthening of the pelvic floor for proper muscle relaxation. In the clinic, I see post-partum mamas every day who present with tension in their pelvic floors and lack of proper lengthening. This can lead to painful sex, tailbone pain, and dysfunction with bowel or bladder. If you focus on breathing using your diaphragm, every time you inhale, your pelvic floor gets good practice lengthening. Then, as you exhale, the diaphragm and pelvic floor move back upwards. Why does this matter? Well, let's say you delivered your baby and now you leak a little urine every time you sneeze. We need to re-educate the pelvic floor muscles on how to properly contract (see Chapters 8 and 9), and the first step is gaining the proper upward movement of the pelvic floor on exhalation.

Bear with the physiology, we're almost there.

As NICU mamas, we often live in "fight, flight, or freeze." I'm sure I was in this for at least the first three months of our NICU stay, and then it returned when we came home. Our brain's job is to keep us safe and alert us about danger. Babies in isolettes and not in our arms? The brain senses danger. Alarms? Danger. Scalp IV's? Danger. Bilirubin lights? Danger. You get the idea. If our brain stays in this state all of the time in the NICU, our hearts race, our breathing is rapid and shallow, our pupils dilate, and blood is rushed to our arms and legs so that we can run or fight to protect ourselves. The blood then rushes away from areas our brain deems less important. We have trouble with memory, learning, making decisions, and digestion because our brains do not consider these important at the moment. How do you turn this system down and try to tell your brain that you are safe? Begin with diaphragmatic breathing. As your breathing slows, your heart rate will slow and your nervous system will begin to calm. The more you do this, the better you can think, respond, learn, sleep, and digest. Your immunity improves which is essential for NICU parents. Your body can better heal from vaginal delivery or c-section. You will have an improved ability to understand what the medical team is telling you, and you will be more equipped to make important decisions.

If you are able to have kangaroo care with your baby (holding your little one skin to skin), you can practice diaphragmatic breathing during this time. Kangaroo care has been shown to stabilize babies' heart rates and regulate their breathing, while also increasing milk production for the mother. In the world of the NICU, we can feel lost and there are so many things we can't control. Practicing deep, slow breathing is a way you can help both you AND your baby with just a simple breathing technique, and the results in both of you can be profound.

Questions

1. After watching in the mirror or on your phone, where do you notice expansion during breathing? Do you seem to breathe more from your chest or your diaphragm?

2. Are your breaths short or long? Do you breathe through your nose, mouth, or both?

3. Try the diaphragmatic breathing exercise. How do you feel now?

Chapter 5: Vaginal Delivery Mamas

Because so many babies are delivered each year (4 million in the US alone, 2/3 of which are born vaginally), we tend to overlook and not give enough HUGE respect to what actually happens. Let me give you a few statistics to put vaginal delivery into perspective. This is not written to scare any pregnant mamas out there, but instead to say "you are a total bad ass" to those who have already traveled this journey. C-section mamas, hang in there until the next chapter because, spoiler alert, we are total bad assess, too!

To vaginally deliver a baby, pelvic floor muscles have been shown to stretch up to three times their normal length. Imagine for a moment any other muscle in your body doing this. Picture in your head this happening with your calf or neck muscles. Ouch. Also, after delivery, there is a healing "scab" the size of a dinner plate on your uterus where the placenta was attached. Look around on your body for that irritating little scab you got from a paper cut or maybe even a small scar that needed stitches from when you cut your arm. Now, go back to what I said earlier. Healing area the size of a *dinner plate*. If that doesn't make you respect yourself enough to realize your healing is important, I'm not sure what else could. You deserve to care for yourself and your recovery, and you can do this without compromising the time and attention you give your little one while they lay in their isolette.

First, let's talk about some things you can do to ease immediate post-vaginal delivery pain. If you are further in your post-partum journey, keep reading – if you ever decide to have another baby, this is important information and if not, you can always share it with your sister, best friend, or co-worker.

1. **Ice:** Ice to the perineal region (area between the vaginal and rectal openings) can help to decrease pain and swelling. Ask a friend or family member to quickly make up some frozen pads (padsicles) to drop off – you can find instructions on Pinterest. For your first urination post-delivery, some hospitals provide a lidocaine spray to reduce discomfort.

2. **Bowel movements:** Let's talk about the first (dreaded) bowel movement post-vaginal delivery. If you are already past this point, this information also applies to anyone who has constipation (see Chapter 11) or again – this can be info to share with your newly pregnant BFF. The best thing to do for a pain-free bowel movement is to sit on the toilet in the position that helps the pelvic floor muscles relax. First, we need to elevate the feet. At our clinic, we love, love, love a product called the Squatty Potty which is a 7–8-inch stepstool made specifically for optimal bowel movement position, but I've also had patients put their feet up on toddler step stools, milk crates, and more. When you put your feet on a step stool, your knees go up above your hips and this helps the pelvic floor muscles let go so that a bowel movement is easier. Also, it provides the poop more of a straight route to exit as opposed to going around sort of a corner, like it has to with your feet on the floor. Some of our patients take a Squatty Potty with them to the hospital for after delivery (they make a travel version), but another easy option is to turn over a trash can and place your feet up on that. Next, lean your forearms over onto your thighs and as you gently bear down, blow out as if you are blowing out birthday candles. This pushes the air out, reducing the pressure down on your newly-healing pelvic floor.

3. **Abdominal binder:** I like to recommend that patients purchase an abdominal binder (a simple Velcro support that you can get inexpensively online) that you wear when you are up and around for a few weeks following your delivery to help the connective

tissue lay down properly as your now non-pregnant body begins to try to figure out how to return to its previous position (I'm not talking weight loss, ladies, I'm talking connective tissue – the sticky stuff that holds all of our organs together and holds our organs to our bony skeleton). This is just for when you are up and about, such as *when you are walking around in the NICU.* Make sure it is on at a comfortable level of tightness and isn't pushing pressure down toward your pelvic floor. You can ask a nurse to help you, but be aware you might have to bring your own as only some hospitals provide them. (Hey ladies reading this on bedrest – "add to cart" now!) You can usually discontinue using the abdominal binder after a few weeks and progress to support garments as needed (see below). If you choose not to use a binder or find them uncomfortable, I would recommend at least using a support garment (Check out #4!)

4. **Support garments:** If you are recovering from vaginal varicosities or just feel like a little extra support in the vaginal/abdominal area would be helpful, see the Resources section for my favorite post-partum support garments. There is a huge range of items to choose from depending on how much money you want to spend and how much support you feel you need. Options include post-partum leggings with perineal and belly support, belly bands, post-partum shorts, special underwear with extra support, and simple non-pregnancy related, high-waisted leggings.

Often with vaginal deliveries, women experience tearing or have an episiotomy. According to the American Academy of Obstetrics and Gynecology (ACOG), 53-79% of women experience tearing during vaginal delivery. Vaginal tears are given a description of Grades 1-4. It is okay if you do not know the grade of your tear (I often find this when patients had a delivery many years ago); while it does provide helpful information about your recovery process, you can treat it without knowing the details.

Vaginal tearing most often occurs in the perineum, the area between the lowest part of your vaginal opening and your rectum. Tears can go straight down from the bottom of the vaginal opening or they can angle to one side. Tears can also occur in the labia.

Grade 1: Extends from the vagina into the perineum; affects the first layer of superficial tissue (not muscle)

Grade 2: Extends from your vagina into the perineum; affects superficial tissue as well as into the muscular layer

Grade 3: Extends from your vagina to your anus and anal sphincter muscles; typically, involves superficial and muscular layers

Grade 4: Extends from the vagina through the perineum and anal sphincter; then tears into the rectum. This is the most severe level of tearing.

The owner of the clinic where I work has a great analogy for vaginal tears. Grade 1 and 2 tears are comparable to a simple shoulder arthroscopic surgery while Grade 3 and 4 tears are more comparable to a rotator cuff repair. If you're more of a knee person, think of Grades 1 and 2 as a meniscus tear and Grades 3 and 4 as an ACL reconstruction. While all are very important to rehab, treatment for the more severe tears is absolutely essential – and not addressed enough.

Some patients may have an episiotomy during delivery in which the perineum is cut to allow the baby to be delivered. While this used to be standard practice, they are not used as frequently anymore however there are still instances where they are performed in order to safely deliver the baby. Similar to tears, it is very important to rehab after an episiotomy.

Prior to your six-week follow-up, you do not want to apply pressure to the scar itself as it needs time to heal. Begin with slow, relaxing belly breathing while trying to imagine the pelvic floor and vaginal region lengthening and relaxing every time you inhale. This can be done sitting right next to your baby's isolette or even while you are holding your little one. You can perform gentle soft tissue massage to the inner thighs and back of the hips. Assess and correct your posture (return to Chapter 1 for posture information and ways to complete soft tissue massage). At around six weeks, follow-up with your OB-GYN, and she will tell you if your scar is healed enough to proceed with touch and mobilization.

Once released by your OB-GYN, I progress scar mobilization differently depending on how much discomfort the patient is having. To begin, I encourage patients to breathe, release any tightness in the muscles nearby, and begin desensitization of the scar. To do this, find items of different textures (clean and soft t-shirt, a tissue, a cotton ball, etc.). Place these items on the scar so the nerves can begin to feel different textures once again. Do not rub with these items! Simply touch.

I also have patients begin to move the scar by gathering the tissue *around* it instead of mobilizing the scar itself (you can usually start this technique prior to your six-week follow-up since you are working around the scar as opposed to directly on it). Place your thumb and forefinger on either side of your scar and gently gather (not pinch!) the tissue together. Once the tissue is gathered, shift your thumb and finger to one side, pulling the tissue in that direction, then move the tissue back to the other side. Eventually, as tenderness decreases and you are released by your OB-GYN, mamas can then progress to touching right on their scar and massaging gentle circles clockwise and counterclockwise to make sure there are no adhesions that keep the tissue stuck down, reducing natural movement and potentially causing pain throughout the day or with intercourse. You may also then complete the thumb stretch assessment/treatment as described in Chapter 13, treating what you find. If you are still having pain at your scar or vaginal region after trying these options, I would highly suggest seeing a pelvic floor physical therapist.

Okay, so now let's think beyond the scar to the muscles beneath. Remember, these muscles have supported your growing and changing body for the entire pregnancy and then stretched three times their normal length during delivery. Tears that are Grade 2 or higher involve tearing into these muscles. This can lead to pelvic floor muscles that are too tight, too weak, or both. Give yourself a couple weeks to heal after your delivery and then you can gently start assessing how your pelvic floor muscles feel (and remember, if you are twenty years beyond your vaginal delivery, you can still start with this)! Begin by noticing if your pelvic floor muscles feel relaxed while quietly sitting or lying down. They should not feel like they are holding back urine unless you are actually on your way to the bathroom. Inhale using your diaphragm, expanding your belly. Try to notice if your pelvic floor lengthens (for example, if you are sitting, it should feel like the muscles move down toward the chair, but keep in mind, this is a very small movement). Exhale through your mouth and feel if the muscles return to neutral. If you don't feel much yet, don't worry – many mamas don't! Keep practicing. If everything feels good, you can try a very simple strengthening exercise.

Super gentle pelvic floor muscle contraction

Inhale using your diaphragm and feel your pelvic floor lengthen. Exhale through your mouth and very gently contract your pelvic floor by pretending you are picking up a blueberry with your vagina. Remember, it's a blueberry so don't try to squeeze super hard. Then release your muscles and focus on putting the blueberry *all the way back down* (super important)! How does this feel? There should be no pain, and you should be able to feel the difference between contraction and relaxation. Begin with only 10 contractions each day. Stop if you notice pain or if you have any other signs that your pelvic floor may be stuck in the "clenched" position such as difficulty with bowel movements, urinary frequency, hesitant urine stream, or just a feeling that you can't let go. In these cases, proceed to Chapter 13 to focus on getting the pelvic floor to relax before focusing on strengthening.

After a vaginal delivery, you will commonly follow-up with your OB-GYN at 6 weeks. At this point, she will most likely release you for everything – sex, CrossFit, running a marathon, everything. Do not, I repeat DO NOT, jump directly back into any of these things! Also, do not fall into the incorrect assumption that all of the other post-partum women out there in the world are immediately doing these things. Your tissue does not fully heal until 12 weeks post-partum, and we encourage all of our mamas to wait until at least this time before doing any high-level activities, and that is AFTER you have properly rehabbed yourself and your shocked musculoskeletal system. Continue reading to see how you can do this while never leaving your baby's side, but at this point, I just want to emphasize that just because you are released, you should not jump back into activity and you should not believe that this is at all the "normal" – because it is, most emphatically, not.

I think the most important suggestion I have about vaginal deliveries is to recognize what an enormous and amazing feat this was for your body. It doesn't matter if you delivered at twenty-three weeks or forty-one weeks, you literally pushed a baby through your vagina into the world. I think many of the patients I treat and women I know don't stop and think about how incredible this is because, it's true, millions of women do this every year – but that doesn't make it ANY less extraordinary.

Questions

1. Did you have a vaginal delivery? If so, describe what happened and how you felt.

2. How did you feel like you recovered after your vaginal delivery? Do you know if you had any tearing or an episiotomy? (If you aren't sure and you want to know, contact your OB's office or medical records).

3. If you had a vaginal delivery, how did it compare to what you expected? What was the same and what was different?

4. What advice would you give a friend who is preparing to have a vaginal delivery?

Chapter 6:
C-section Mamas

Many NICU mamas, myself included, deliver in an emergency situation which means that often the fastest and safest way to bring the baby into the world is via c-section. Let's talk about c-section in general for a minute and then we'll get real for our NICU mamas.

As a pelvic health physical therapist, I treat post-partum women every day following their c-sections. Mamas, they cut through seven (SEVEN!) layers of tissue when they do this procedure. Because of the fact that this surgery delivers a baby, all of the attention (by medical providers and often ourselves) is then shifted to the baby. Can you imagine any other situation when someone had a surgery that left them with a six-inch long incision and then never really addressed it again? Let me bring this into perspective as a physical therapist....

If someone has a rotator cuff repair, typical recovery may start with six weeks during which time the arm is in an immobilizer so it may heal. Then, there may be another four weeks of activity that is restricted to avoid lifting any weight, even 2 pounds. Then, often around 3-4 months post-op, the patient may be cleared to begin lifting light weights and during ALL of this time, they are attending physical therapy 2-3 times/week.

Let's do the math.

That is approximately thirty-six physical therapy visits to recover from a rotor cuff surgery.

Now, here is the typical recovery from a c-section (remember, surgery that cuts through seven layers of tissue).

Return to the OB for a six-week follow-up. Resume all activities. ALL. Intercourse. Running. HIIT workouts. Ladies – NO!

Also, remember, that's a "typical" c-section (never really a typical one, but hang with me for a second). Let's take this and think about a NICU delivery.

I had an emergency c-section and then basically put it out of my mind – I didn't have time. I know many of you can relate to this. My babies were having spells of apnea and bradycardia (decreased oxygen and drops in heart rate) every 1-2 minutes, and my attention was on brain hemorrhages, blood transfusions, and infections. My brain was so preoccupied, I actually had less post-op pain (see Chapter 14), but it also led me to completely ignore proper c-section rehab which is a HUGE reason why I am writing this book in the first place.

You can properly rehab your c-section and not lose ANY time with your baby. You can also properly rehab your c-section without missing any new updates or information in the NICU. As a pelvic floor physical therapist, I have taken the suggestions we give all of our c-section mamas and catered them specifically to a recovering mom who is immersed in the world of neonatal intensive care.

<u>**What you can start right away**</u>

1. **Diaphragmatic breathing (review from Chapter 4):** You can literally start this in your hospital bed. Place a hand on your abdomen or place a hand beneath each side of the rib cage. Inhale through your nose slowly (for at least two seconds) and focus on expanding your ribs out and your abdomen toward the ceiling. This should be pain-free so do not expand to the point of pain in your new incision. Then, exhale through your mouth slowly for 2-4 seconds and let your belly go back down. Your ribs should also come back down. Mamas, the more you can do this, the better. Every time you breathe using your diaphragm, it causes your pelvic floor to descend and RELAX. This helps avoid future post-partum pelvic floor

muscle tension issues such as painful sex. Also, when you slow your breathing and focus on your diaphragm, it calms your body, bringing you out of the "fight, flight, or freeze" response that we become stuck in as NICU mamas. This can lead to an entire cascade of improvements in your body (this stuff is my favorite - see Chapter 14).

2. **Gentle abdominal tissue massage:** This first sentence is super important: do not massage directly on your c-section scar for the first 6 weeks until released by your physician. It needs to heal; we are going to begin doing work AROUND the scar, not directly on it. While diaphragmatic breathing can begin as soon as you are up to it, I would begin this tissue work around 1-2 weeks post-partum (but remember, keep this gentle, pain-free, and away from your scar). Begin right beneath your ribs. Take two fingers and gently press into the tissue just a little – remember, this should never be painful. Slowly and gently, glide the tissue from the outside in toward the middle. Then, move down a little bit and move that tissue the same way. Work the entire tummy area stopping a few inches above your scar (or earlier, if you start to feel discomfort). You can also perform this technique below the scar. The point of this technique is to get that tissue moving right away so the scar heals properly and does not develop adhesions beneath it which can lead to future pain, postural dysfunction, and difficulty properly activating your core muscles. And mamas – this can be done *sitting or standing next to your baby's isolette!* You do not need to lie down, you do not need to remove your shirt (just sneak your hand under it) ... you can do this while being RIGHT THERE with your little one, losing no time with him at all.

3. **Abdominal binder (this is a review from the vaginal delivery chapter):** At our clinic, we like to recommend that patients purchase an abdominal binder that you wear when you are up and around for a few weeks following your c-section to help the

connective tissue lay down properly as your body begins to try to figure out how to return to its previous position. This is just for when you are up and about, such as *when you are walking around in the NICU.* Make sure it is on at a comfortable level of tightness and does not put pressure down on the pelvic floor. You can always ask a nurse to help you, but be aware you might have to bring your own as only some hospitals provide them. This can be helpful whether you delivered at 23 weeks or 40. Typically, our patients wear the binder for a few weeks, progressing to supportive leggings or belly bands when they feel ready (see Resources).

4. **Bowel movements after delivery:** Yikes, am I right? I avoided a lot of rehab after my c-section, but we all know a bowel movement has to happen whether your baby is at home or in the NICU so let's talk about it. If I am talking to a new mom (or anyone else who wants to have better bowel movements), I tell them about a product I love called the Squatty Potty. It's a little stool that fits right beside your toilet and when you put your feet up on it, your knees are above your hips. This position helps the pelvic floor muscles relax (needed to allow poop to leave the body) and it creates an easier path for the poop to travel. Place your feet up on the stool, lean your forearms onto your thighs, and blow out while you gently bear down. This helps release the air pressure out of your body; otherwise, it can become trapped and push down on your pelvic floor muscles and pelvic organs as well as out on your healing belly. Pelvic floor physical therapists can get *really* excited about Squatty Potties because we love them so much. So, at home – get a Squatty Potty. But what about your first bowel movement in the hospital? Plus, later, being a NICU mama, you're away from home a LOT - so what can you do if you need to go in that hospital bathroom down the hall? We have definitely had new mamas bring a Squatty Potty into their mother/baby hospital room (they even have a travel one), but many NICU mamas don't have the luxury of packing a hospital bag. If you are in your hospital room or the bathroom in your NICU

hallway is single-stall, turn a trash can over on the side and elevate your feet on that. The next best option is to lean forward, place your forearms on your legs, and blow out while you gently bear down.

5. **Proper movement to get out of bed:** Do not sit straight up out of bed – this is going to hurt, trust me. Instead, do what physical therapists call the "log roll." If you are in your bed (hospital or at home, you'll want to continue this for a while and it's really how we should all be getting up anyway since it is good for our backs), roll to one side first and then use your arms to help push you up to the seated position. You can also grab a pillow and gently press it against your c-section scar as you do this for added support.

6. **Pillow support:** That same pillow I just mentioned above? Keep it nearby in your bed. If you feel a cough, sneeze, or laugh coming on, brace the pillow against your abdomen to help reduce pain.

7. **Abdominal stabilization:** As soon as you feel comfortable, you can begin to gently activate your lower abdominals when moving around for support. This is a very mild contraction and used only to eliminate pain with movement. If pain increases by gently activating your abdominals, it is likely too early and you need to wait. By a few weeks post-partum, you can begin to work this into a very gentle zip-it-up exercise. Inhale with your diaphragm, exhale and gently zip those lower abs up from the pubic bone to the belly button. Hold for 5 seconds and then release. As always, this is general information only and should not be substituted for any advice your doctor has given you about using your abdominals after surgery.

8. **Scar desensitization:** If you find that your scar is very sensitive, try gently touching around it (before fully healed) and on it (once healed) with various textures to begin to calm the nerves. Take a soft cotton ball and just set it on the scar. Try a warm washcloth, a

soft blanket, or just your hand. Do not rub with these items, just touch.

9. **Begin a walking program:** For the first couple weeks, focus on breathing, proper movement, getting sleep when you can, hydrating, and nourishing your body with warm, easy to digest foods (don't worry, I take real life into consideration – see Chapter 7). Once you begin to feel a bit better, you can start to work on a gentle walking program. If your little one is in the NICU, you can use the hospital hallways. You can always take a lap around the parking lot before or after visiting (or when you need a much-deserved break for some fresh air). If you are struggling with being overwhelmed with the NICU experience (and what NICU parent hasn't experienced this at some point), *it is okay* to go into the hospital a half hour later so you can walk around your neighborhood for both your physical and mental health. *It is okay* to leave the hospital a half hour earlier to go home and walk a (slow at first) loop with your neighbor. I know I struggled with leaving the hospital and doing anything for myself however when I look back now, I realize taking more breaks would have recharged my internal battery so much for those inevitable tough moments in the NICU.

   <u>**A general guide**</u>

   - Remember that everyone is different and the most important thing is to listen to your own body.
   - For the first week, work on a few minutes, several times a day, likely around the NICU.
   - By week two, work up to 5-8 minutes a couple times each day (this may very well be to and from the hospital parking lot if you have been discharged and your little one is still in the NICU).
   - By week three, work on 8-10 minutes a couple times a day and from here, slowly add a few minutes each week as it feels comfortable.

10. **Gentle pelvic floor movement:** Inhale using your diaphragm, exhale and gently activate the pelvic floor by imagining you are picking up a blueberry with your vagina. Then, *fully relax it back down.* The goal of this is not to do a lot of Kegels and build up strength – remember, too much pelvic floor muscle tension can be very common. Instead, the goal is to encourage natural movement of the pelvic floor, working through the full range of motion, and to notice if there are any concerns. Begin with 10 contractions a day. If you have difficulty with either muscle relaxation or contraction, discuss with your OB and ask for a referral to pelvic floor PT.

<u>What you can do a little later</u>

1. **Scar massage:** Around six weeks, new mamas usually have their follow-up appointment with the OB-GYN and as long as the scar is healing well and there are no open areas, you usually get the all-clear to begin scar massage right on the scar. Please note – you may not be told to do scar massage because again, you are usually just released for any and all activity without much guidance. Feel free to bring it up to your doctor or ask for a referral to pelvic floor physical therapy to be guided by a trained professional. Now that the scar is healed, the gentle tissue massage you were performing above and below your scar can now be very gently completed right over your scar, avoiding pain. I recommend patients massage gentle circles clockwise and counterclockwise above, below, and on the scar. Be sure to move the tissue in all directions: up, down, and to each side. You may find that your tissue moves well, but do not be concerned if you feel like the tissue is tight or lumpy – that is why we are doing this technique. If you find your scar is very sensitive, focus on circles above and below the scar while working on desensitization techniques on the scar itself until it feels better.

It is also normal at this point for the scar to be fairly numb. Nerves are notoriously slow healers so this numbness can continue for a while (we're talking, like a year). Some women will have a little bit of numbness that remains, but for many mamas, the feeling comes back, but it can be a slow process. Your scar commonly looks raised for a while (my patients often ask if it will stay "puffy") and over time, this will improve and usually, this will go down to where it is hardly visible. Scar massage can help move this along, but do not push hard in order to reduce the puffiness – this comes with time and healing, and irritating it could make things worse.

2. **Advance walking:** If walking has been progressing well, helps you relieve stress, and improves your stamina, you can continue to add a few minutes each day. I would highly advise waiting to return to running or high-intensity exercise until approximately 12 weeks post-partum and more specifically, after being evaluated by a qualified pelvic health physical therapist.

3. **Pool work:** If you have access to one, getting into a pool can be amazing for c-section mamas (*once your scar is fully healed so you do not risk infection*). Work on gentle walking (forward, sideways, backwards), heel raises, mini squats, and bicycling your legs while floating on a couple pool noodles. Keep everything pain-free! This may sound like a large time commitment away from the NICU, but even once a week could help.

4. **Advance stabilization exercises:** Begin with the zip-it-up exercise. If everything is feeling good, see Chapter 16 for additional exercises to complete while progressing back into activity.

Questions

1. Did you have a c-section? If so, describe what you can remember about your surgery.

2. Have you ever looked at or touched your scar? How do you feel about doing that?

3. Was your c-section planned or unplanned? How did you feel when you found out you were going to have a c-section?

4. How was your recovery for the first few weeks after your surgery?

5. What advice would you give a friend who is preparing to have a c-section?

Chapter 7:
Fueling Your Body

Let's do our plan versus NICU reality again. Okay, let's imagine your healthy, plump full-term baby comes home from the hospital with you after a day or so of recovery (cue the mental image we all had in our heads of mama and new baby being pushed out the front entrance of the hospital in a wheelchair surrounded by balloons and teddy bears). At night, you pull out the freezer meals you prepared knowing when you were going to go into labor (40 weeks, of course) and heat up a nice, healthy, home-cooked meal that is nutritious and healing following your delivery, supercharging you to take care of your new baby.

*Spoiler alert: this isn't actually how it ends up going for any new mom, let's be real, but we can all imagine it, right?

I went into the hospital on antepartum at 22 weeks, 5 days gestation, and from then until I delivered, my husband and I ate hospital food (not complaining, ours was actually super good). I had the babies at 24 weeks, 1 day gestation, and our friends and family stepped up like champions. They stocked our freezer, cleaned our house, and cared for our pets. When we would come home from our days in the NICU, we could easily throw something someone had so kindly made us in the oven. So, if someone asks what they can do for you? FOOD. Ideally, (pelvic health PT coming out here), food that nourishes your gut as you heal, specifically warm, healthy foods like broth-based soups with cooked vegetables that are easy to digest.

Here's the thing, though. Some of us don't have loved ones nearby. And, as in our case, our babies were in the NICU for 122 days, and I did not want to continue asking friends and family for food (though I should have and strongly encourage you to do this). As I prepared to write this chapter, I sat and tried really hard to remember what we ate during that entire time, and I have absolutely no recollection. I can't remember a single trip to the grocery store although I'm sure I must have gone weekly or so.

As in most NICUs, we were not allowed to have snacks or drinks in our babies' rooms however there was a parent room down the hall. I remember going down there to chug some water at times. I never once ate a meal downstairs in the cafeteria because I couldn't bear spending any of my hospital time away from the babies' rooms in part because I wanted to spend time with them and didn't want to miss anything and in part, I now realize, because of the guilt I was carrying for feeling like it was my fault that they were there in the first place.

After a few weeks, I went back to work for four hours each morning to see a few patients so I could save my twelve weeks of maternity leave for after the babies came home. I would see my patients then strap on my hands-free pumping bra in my treatment room and pump, write patient notes, and eat a sandwich all at the same time. Good for efficiency, not so much for gut healing and giving my body what it needed to take on the NICU later that day.

Let me pause here for one second. If you are reading this beyond your NICU journey and realize this is what you did the whole time, *it's okay.* That was me, too. Take this information and use it NOW as you care for little kids which is certainly a challenge all its own. If you are a current NICU mama and you catch yourself multi-tasking to make it through, *that's okay, too.* I firmly believe the best way to make it through a NICU journey is day by day or even hour by hour (or minute by minute in those early days). So, the last thing I want you to do is beat yourself up if you are starving and your lunch is chips in your car as you drive to the hospital. It happens to all of us and any fuel is better than nothing. However, when you can, use these tips to try to make nourishing your body a bit easier so that you can be the strongest, healthiest mom you can be to the little one who needs you so much.

1. **Grocery pick-up:** I'm not sure this was a thing eight years ago when my kids were in the NICU, but it's available at almost all grocery stores now, usually free or for a small fee unless you want delivery (which is even more awesome, but may cost you a touch more). You can make your grocery list and even order it from your phone or computer as you sit in your baby's room. NICU babies sleep a lot and often there is not much you can do between cares, especially in those early stages when holding your baby may be limited. I know I spent a lot of time sitting in that mint green recliner and that would have been the perfect time to make an order.

   Now, what to order? If you feel that realistically, you might do some chopping and make freezer meals on a weekend for the week, that's amazing and I highly recommend it. Don't feel pressure to commit that much time, though, as you can make quick, easy, and healthy meals on week nights if you need to. Think healthy, but also simple – soups, stir fries, chicken, fish. You might even want to invest in a meal delivery service where the meals come dropped off on your porch and you just have to follow some simple directions.

2. **When friends, family, or neighbors ask what they can do, don't be shy to ask for food**. Even better, ask one close friend to start a meal train so that the food keeps coming. Think warm, nourishing foods like soups and casseroles that are easy to heat up quickly for when you come home from the hospital and just want to drop straight into bed from exhaustion, but your body – and your *baby* – need you to have strength and fuel. People do really want to help you when your baby is in the NICU and often bringing food is the only way they know how so allowing them to make you food helps both you *and them.*

3. **Water:** It sounds so simple, right? Yet, I can't even begin to tell you how many conversations I have each week with my patients about the importance of water and how many times I hear people admit that they are not drinking enough. Often, my new moms are my

exception as they know they need to hydrate well for breast feeding. If you're like me, though, it becomes tricky when you can't drink by your baby's isolette. I highly recommend investing in whatever stainless steel water bottle you love the most, filling it up first thing in the morning, and drinking from it when you can. You may not be able to drink right at your baby's bedside so be sure to drink a good 8-10 ounces when you wake up, drink with your breakfast, sip on the drive to the hospital, and it is okay – full permission here – to step away from your baby for a few minutes to go wherever your hospital has for NICU parents to eat, drink, and relax. Drink some water, toss back some almonds, close your eyes and do some deep breathing – and then you can go right back to your baby, but your body will be better able to serve you and your little one after those five minutes of self-care.

4. **Healthy snacks:** I recommend avoiding processed foods in favor of ones that are more nutrient-dense which can lead to improved tissue healing (remember you just had a baby!) and less inflammation. Create your own trail mix with a mixture of nuts. Make a big bag so that you can grab two handfuls, toss them in a baggie, and stick them in your NICU bag for the day. Another favorite of mine? Energy balls! You can make a wide variety, but my go-to is a mixture of oatmeal, peanut butter, honey, coconut, flax seed (to help out those bowel movements), a little vanilla, and dark chocolate chips. Simply mix it up and roll them into little balls, storing them in the fridge. If you have a cooler that you use to transport your breast milk, it's easy to stash a couple of these in a baggie in there. Instant protein, calories, and energy with minimal preservatives and processing (plus, they taste amazing and we can all use a little peanut butter-dark chocolate when trying to make it through the turbulence of the NICU).

5. **Warm, nourishing foods:** Again, think soups, chicken, fish, or vegetables. Remember, you just delivered a baby and your tissues

need to heal. Collagen specifically is very good to promote tissue healing. An excellent source of this is bone broth, which is a broth that is similar to chicken or beef broth that is boiled longer and a little bit differently. I actually think drinking a small cup of warm bone broth by itself is tasty however I have had some patients who don't like it straight. You can use it as a base for soups (think good old chicken noodle), and if you still aren't loving the taste, make the soup with half bone broth and half chicken broth. Do be aware of high sodium content in some bone broths and choose accordingly. There are also collagen powders and supplements. As with any supplement, especially if you are breast feeding, run this by your doctor or your child's pediatrician before beginning to take them. Warm, cooked vegetables are nourishing and easier to digest than raw veggies so add these when you can.

6. **Calories, mamas, calories:** We've all heard "you're eating for two" when you're pregnant (or more, if you're having multiples!), but what a lot of women don't realize is that if you are breast feeding (don't forget, pumping IS breast feeding), you actually need more calories now than you did when you were pregnant. This becomes even trickier for the NICU mama who cannot necessarily just sit and snack when in her baby's room. Make sure foods and snacks are nutrient dense. Think avocados (you can buy single-serving avocado spread to make transport easier), nuts, hearty soups, animal proteins, and cooked vegetables. Unless otherwise directed by your physician, now is not the time to restrict calories in order to start losing the baby weight. You have to feed your body so that your milk (should you choose to breast feed or pump) can nourish your baby.

7. **Mindful eating:** Basically, this is the opposite of what I remember doing (and if you're past your NICU stay and this was you, too, no worries – you can focus on mindful eating now, especially during post-NICU times of stress). What I did: shove a sandwich in my

mouth while I was pumping so I could get everything done before I drove to the NICU. I never tasted a thing – I think maybe I chewed a few times? Mindful eating: Slow down and don't multi-task. I know this feels practically impossible during the rushing about that often goes along with a NICU stay, so don't expect to be perfect at this every time and that is completely okay. When you can, though, try to pause and slow down. Sit at the table, set your phone down, and slowly chew each bite. Sometimes it helps to eat with your fork or spoon in your non-dominant hand if you have trouble not rushing (or at the very least, focus on putting it down between each bite). Close your eyes if necessary. Focus on the smell and taste of the food. Not only will this help your digestion, it will also help bring you down out of "fight, flight, or freeze" which will help your sleep, focus, muscle tension, and ability to learn and form new memories.

8. **Inflammatory foods vs non-inflammatory foods:** When most of us think of inflammation, we might think of the time we rolled our ankle, it got puffy and purple, and we elevated it with an ice pack to reduce the swelling. In fact, inflammation can result from more than just an acute injury. Certain foods can actually lead to increased inflammation while others can *decrease* it. Now, imagine you delivered a baby (whether this has been two weeks ago or two years ago). This can be a vaginal delivery or a c-section; healing is required either at the abdomen for a c-section, at the perineum for any vaginal tearing, and for everyone, where the placenta was attached to the uterus. Prioritize foods that reduce inflammation; think blueberries, pineapple, basil, oregano, turmeric, dark leafy greens, olive oil, and fatty fish. Reduce your intake of foods that increase inflammation which include alcohol, sugar, dairy, gluten, artificial sweeteners, and soy.

Questions

1. Whether you are a current NICU mama or a NICU mama veteran, how would you describe your diet?

2. What is one thing you are doing well regarding your diet (think about food, beverages, and habits around eating)?

3. What are some ways you would like to improve?

4. Write one goal for the habit you would like to change first.

Chapter 8:
Bladder, Bladder, What's the Matter?

Common, but not normal.

Every pelvic floor physical therapist nods her head because this is what we tell all of our patients. Leakage of urine is common, but it is not normal and it is NOT something you should just accept because you've had a baby. I cannot tell you how many patients I've had over the years who were surprised when their doctors sent them to physical therapy to help their leaking. They just figured that they had a baby, and it was normal to pee a little afterward. Yes, it happens often, but NO, it's doesn't have to be permanent.

Stress incontinence is when you leak urine when a pressure pushes down on your bladder. So, these are the mamas who leak when they sneeze, cough, laugh, run, and jump. Urge incontinence is when suddenly, you have to go really badly and you just can't make it in time. Mixed incontinence is when you have both. While many people associate leakage with pregnant or post-partum women, in my clinic we see males and females of all age groups. We see young kids who leak, women of all ages, and men, commonly after prostate procedures such as prostatectomy. Leakage can be a small amount when just a couple drops wet your underwear or it can be enough that you have to wear an incontinence pad (side note – if this is you at this point, be sure to use a pad specifically for urine NOT a menstrual pad).

The best thing about addressing this? All of the simple techniques you need to do can be done right by your baby's side.

A little pelvic floor muscle review so this all makes sense. Your pelvic floor is made up of fourteen different muscles that begin around your pubic bone in the front, travel underneath you (like a hammock), and then attach around your tailbone in the back. There are three layers of these muscles, and they serve multiple purposes which include bowel and bladder continence, support of your pelvic organs, sexual functions such as orgasm, and core stability.

During pregnancy, there is increased pressure on the pelvic floor due to the weight of the baby, uterus, and placenta. This is why women who deliver via c-section are not immune to pelvic floor dysfunction. If you do have a vaginal delivery, these pelvic floor muscles stretch up to three times their resting length. When you imagine what happens to these muscles during delivery, it's easy to understand how in the post-partum period, they might not contract appropriately due to decreased strength, endurance, and coordination. Now, imagine if you have a big sneeze. The intra-abdominal pressure from the sneeze pushes down on the bladder which is partially full of urine (as it is supposed to be, that's it's job), but since the pelvic floor muscles either don't quite remember how to squeeze or they try but they are just too weak, the urine travels from the bladder through the urethra right on out of your body without getting stopped by your pelvic floor. It could also be that the pelvic floor muscles are gripping too hard so that when you sneeze, they are unable to squeeze any further. This can also lead to leakage.

Now, in addition to a baby in the NICU, you have pee in your underwear.

So, let's fix it!

Remember diaphragmatic breathing? Quick reminder – in through your nose for two seconds expanding your belly and ribs, out through your mouth for four seconds while letting them come back down. We are going to learn how to find your pelvic floor muscles and re-teach them to contract properly, using this breathing technique to help us. Here we go. The cueing may sound funny, but I promise you, it works.

Pelvic floor muscle contractions (aka Kegels) done RIGHT!

1. Inhale through your nose, using your diaphragm (belly and ribs expand, not the chest).
2. Exhale out through your mouth and – here's the key – pretend like you are picking up a blueberry with your vagina. (Pause to allow the reader to giggle a little. But again, I promise you, it works). Don't let other muscles, such as your glutes or abdominals, kick in to help out. Then, *fully relax* (this is key).
3. Repeat this nice and slow, allowing plenty of time to relax after each repetition.
4. If you're not loving the blueberry cue, you can also imagine sucking up a smoothie through your vagina. Again, a quirky food analogy, but there is a point to these two particular cues – it helps you find the proper muscles and avoid compensation from other "helper" muscles such as abdominals and glutes.
5. Start with five reps at a time, 3-4 times a day.
6. There should NEVER be any discomfort. Stop immediately if you have any pain, feel you cannot fully relax your muscles, or develop urinary urgency or frequency.
7. IMPORTANT SIDE NOTE: many years ago, women used to be taught to complete these exercises while trying to stop their urine. Do not do this! Women have short urethras and are prone to bladder infections, and a stop/start flow of urine increases the chance of moving bacteria upstream into the urethra, leading to a UTI.

Pelvic floor muscle endurance contractions

1. Once you feel like you have a handle on the quick contractions, you can mix in some endurance contractions. For some women, they can start this right away and for others, this progression may take weeks. Both of these are fine as long as you listen to your own body and do not try to match anyone else.

2. Inhale through your nose, using your diaphragm (belly expands, not the chest).
3. Exhale out through your mouth and once again, imagine you are picking up a blueberry with your vagina. This time, hold the contraction for 3-5 seconds.
4. Fully relax.
5. In the beginning, some women can only hold for 2-3 seconds, others are in the 5-second range, and others can hold a bit longer. The ultimate goal is 10 seconds, but remember, this may not occur for many months post-partum. Do not pressure yourself to do this too quickly as this could lead to tension and pain. As your endurance holds become longer, you will need to breathe in and out again. Keep squeezing, and don't hold your breath!
6. Once you begin to add the endurance contractions, do a mix of quick and endurance contractions each day. Every situation varies, but begin with 20 total contractions per day (think 2 sets of 5 quick contractions and 2 sets of 5 endurance contractions). Work up to 40-60 contractions each day.
7. Again, there should never be any pain!

The "Knack"

Any time you feel a cough or a sneeze coming on, use the pelvic floor muscles to pick up that imaginary blueberry first! By activating the pelvic floor, you are improving your barrier against leakage, hopefully, stopping it 100% (however, this may take time).

Blow as you go

It's common that when people do some type of exertion (such as lifting something like a heavy laundry basket or weight lifting), they hold their breath. Unless you are a power lifter completing a 1 rep max, we need to do the *opposite*. Always exhale during exertion as it will put less air pressure down on your bladder, pelvic floor, and your recovering abdomen.

Example: Let's say you and your NICU baby are home and you are about to lift your baby in her carseat. Inhale first. Exhale and continue to exhale while you are lifting, releasing all of the air pressure from your abdomen. If you have been leaking during these activities, add a pelvic floor muscle contraction. Inhale, exhale and pick up a blueberry. Continue to exhale and hold the blueberry while you lift.

Awareness of dietary irritants

Certain beverages and foods can irritate the bladder and increase your chances of leakage. Be aware of the most common culprits:

- Caffeine (coffee, soda, tea)
- Alcohol
- Citrus juices (orange juice, grapefruit juice, cranberry juice, etc.)
- Artificial sweeteners
- Spicy foods (for some)
- Tomato-based products (for some)

Be aware of what you are drinking and make sure you are drinking plenty of water. This can be hard when your child is in the NICU since water bottles may not be allowed in the room so focus on good water intake driving to the NICU, in the parent room, and driving home. Don't try to catch up right before bed as this will likely lead to you waking frequently at night to urinate. Limit irritants, and if you are going to consume an irritant, make sure you have some water nearby and take multiple sips of water between sips of the irritant. This can help dilute the effect on the bladder which may decrease (but not resolve) the irritant effect.

Remember, some pelvic floor muscles are too tense after pregnancy and delivery. If this is your situation, then I do *not* want you to complete these pelvic floor muscle contractions until we can teach the muscles to fully lengthen. Signs that you might be having pelvic floor muscle tension include pelvic pain, pain with intercourse, a hesitant urine stream, urinary frequency, or difficulty using a tampon or menstrual cup. Also, you might be experiencing pelvic floor muscle tension if you have difficulty relaxing your muscles between contractions. If you feel you may have muscle tension, proceed to Chapter 13 (even if you are not having pain with sex) for some ideas to help improve muscle relaxation prior to beginning these contractions. As always, if you continue to have symptoms, I encourage you to seek help from a pelvic floor physical therapist.

Finally, if leakage primarily occurs during high level activities (such as running or jumping), you can begin here and then progress to Chapter 16 for more information on returning to activity.

Questions

1. Do you ever leak urine? What tends to make this happen? (ex: cough, sneeze, laugh, not making it to the bathroom in time)

2. Evaluate your diet for bladder irritants. What do you notice, and are there any changes you are willing to make?

3. Try a pelvic floor muscle contraction. Do you feel the muscles lift? Can you feel them fully relax?

4. Try engaging the pelvic floor before you cough or sneeze. What do you notice?

5. Pick up a box or laundry basket (or your baby, if you are already home from the NICU) the way you normally do. Put it (or him) down. Then, lift again while blowing out and "picking up a blueberry with your vagina." Is this different than what you were doing before? How does it feel?

Chapter 9:
There's a Bulge in my Vagina: Treating Pelvic Organ Prolapse

So, you're already dealing with a baby in the NICU, which should be enough stress for anyone, but you've also been feeling some pressure in the pelvic region so one day you take a look with a mirror, and…you can *see something* in your vagina that wasn't there before. Or maybe you've been experiencing the odd sensation of having a used tampon in your vagina, and this has moved from annoying to concerning since it just won't go away.

At our clinic, we hear reports like this all the time.

"It feels like my organs are falling out!"

"I can't seem to have an easy bowel movement anymore, and sometimes I have to push with my finger to get it to come out."

"It feels like a baby's head crowning."

"I tried to exercise, but it makes the feeling worse. Now, I'm terrified to move, to pick up my new baby, or chase after my toddler. Will this ever go away???"

First of all, if you are reading this and it does *not* sound familiar, that's awesome and you can jump ahead. Or, keep reading because we can all use additional knowledge about our bodies to keep in our back pocket for future pregnancies or to share with our female friends.

You may have what is called a pelvic organ prolapse. If you want an official diagnosis, you can return to your OB-GYN or see a pelvic floor physical therapist. A prolapse is defined as when one or more of your pelvic organs descend down into the vaginal canal. This can be your bladder (called a cystocele), your uterus (uterine prolapse), your rectum (rectocele), or more than one of these. The simplest way to describe how far the prolapse has descended is by using a grading system. Physicians can do a more detailed evaluation called a POP-Q test which takes multiple measurements, however most patients are happy with the simple grading system below.

Grade 1: Slight prolapse, halfway to the hymen*

Grade 2: Prolapse to around the area of the hymen

Grade 3: Prolapse beyond the hymen to the opening of the vagina

Grade 4: Prolapse beyond the vaginal opening

*The hymen is a layer of tissue that is often broken by the first sexual penetration or use of a tampon. Remnants can be seen near the opening of the vagina.

Yes, it sounds terrifying, but here is the first thing you need to know.

Pelvic organ prolapse (especially Grades 1 and 2) are very prevalent, and it is very common for women to have these levels of prolapse without any symptoms.

The next important thing is that if you are having symptoms, you are not doomed to deal with this pressure for the rest of your life. With pelvic floor physical therapy, studies have shown you can keep your prolapse from getting worse, you can resolve your pelvic floor symptoms (such as the falling-out sensation or the feeling of a stuck tampon), and you can potentially decrease the severity of the prolapse itself. I cannot tell you that by doing these exercises, you can fully resolve your prolapse – surgery is the only way to do that. I can tell you, however, that over the years, I have had many, many patients who have returned to all of their previous activities (including running, jumping, and more), and they no longer have symptoms associated with their prolapses.

The first thing to *immediately* address is avoiding the things that can make prolapse worse. The two primary ways I see in the clinic are straining from constipation and improper lifting. If done incorrectly, both can put a strain on the pelvic floor muscles and lead to increased intra-abdominal pressure in the abdomen that pushes down on the pelvic organs, making prolapse worse.

1. **Proper lifting – "Blow as you go":** Think back to a time when you were lifting something heavy – let's say, you were holding one end of a heavy couch. Try to imagine the lift and how your body moved. Most people, especially when lifting something heavy, do the *opposite* of what should be done. They suck in their breath and hold it while they lift, performing what is called a "Valsalva maneuver." Now get that lifting picture in your head again. If you hold your breath and lift, you close the glottis at the top of your airway so no pressure gets out that way. The pressure will find your weakest link and if that is in the pelvic region, it will push down on the pelvic organs, potentially making the prolapse worse (it can also push out on a poorly controlled abdomen – see chapter on Diastasis Recti).

We need to get this pressure *out*, instead of trapping it in. This will relieve the push down on your pelvic organs and out into your abdomen. We do this by blowing *out* anytime there is exertion. By exhaling during times of exertion, the pressure can be released out through the mouth, relieving the pressure put down on the pelvic floor.

Example #1: Let's go back to lifting one end of a heavy couch (side note – please do not do this post-partum, but we'll use it for illustration and talk about more realistic lifting next). Before lifting the couch, you would want to inhale first and then blow out *while* you lift.

More realistic (I hope) example: Your baby may be in the NICU, but you still have to do laundry (sigh). To pick up that basket full of dirty clothes while protecting your pelvic floor, inhale first then exhale while you lift the basket.

Your baby may not be coming home for a while, but start practicing this technique whenever you do any other types of lifts because once your baby is discharged, you will be picking her up and down all day long, and hopefully, your body will already be reprogrammed to blow each time you pick her up. Babies may start out little (mine were only a pound a half), but six months down the road when they are in those (incredibly heavy) carseats, this technique is vital. Picking up the carseat? Blow out. Lifting a 40-pound bag of dog food? Blow out. Picking up sacks of groceries? Blow out. You get the picture.

Other exertion

This "blow as you go" technique is not just for lifting – think of any exertion that you might do throughout your day. This is especially important during pregnancy and the post-partum period however this should really be done lifelong for proper posture and to protect yourself against pain and dysfunction. Other examples of exertion include:

- Getting out of bed
- Getting up off the floor
- Lifts with rotation (think of picking up a heavy diaper bag and turning to put it in the backseat of your car)
- Standing up out of a chair
- When you return to exercise (see Chapter 16)

2. **Bowel health:** With a prolapse, you want to *avoid all straining.* We talked about how to avoid straining while you lift during your day, but another common time women strain? Trying to have a bowel movement when they are constipated! This straining can apply pressure to the pelvic floor and worsen a prolapse. See Chapter 11 for further information on bowel health, but the first step is good toileting position. For a bowel movement, elevate your feet on a step stool (I love the Squatty Potty), lean your forearms onto your thighs, and as you gently bear down, blow out as if you are blowing out birthday candles. This position will help the pelvic floor to relax so the poop can move through while the blowing out will reduce pressure on your pelvic floor.

Other ideas for prolapse

3. **Propping:** Propping is a super easy technique that you can use to decrease the symptoms of a prolapse. Remember, a prolapse is when the bladder, uterus, rectum, or a combination of these begins to descend downward into the vaginal canal. With propping, we use gravity to help us out to take away this pressure. For this technique, you simply lay on your back with a pillow or two under your hips (not your knees, as I've had some patients accidentally do). This should be comfortable and not cause any pain in your back or anywhere else. By having your hips slightly higher than your chest and shoulders, gravity will help bring the pelvic organs back up the vaginal canal toward their original position.
    - Please note – this technique alone will not resolve the prolapse however if you are feeling a lot of pelvic pressure, it can provide some great relief.

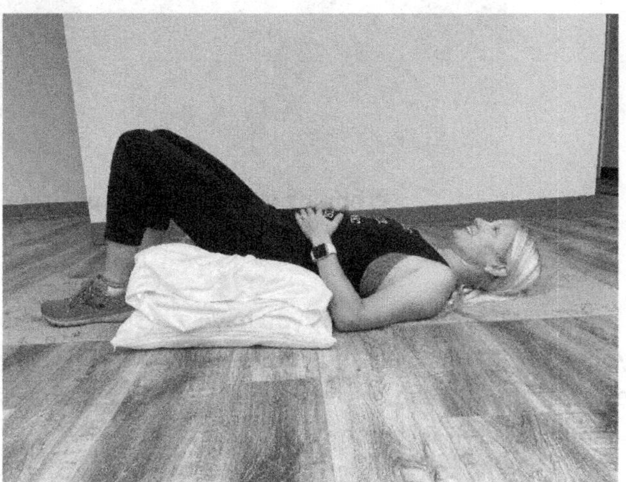

Propping in a bridge position

If you have been told (by either an OB-GYN or a pelvic health physical therapist) that your pelvic organ prolapse is a cystocele (your bladder), this can help you be even more specific with your propping. Your bladder is in front of the vaginal canal so if it is descending, we know it is moving down and *back*. That means that positions such as laying on your belly or being on your hands and knees will encourage the bladder to move forward to the position where it should be. My favorite position for patients with a cystocele is child's pose because this helps the bladder move both forward *and* up.

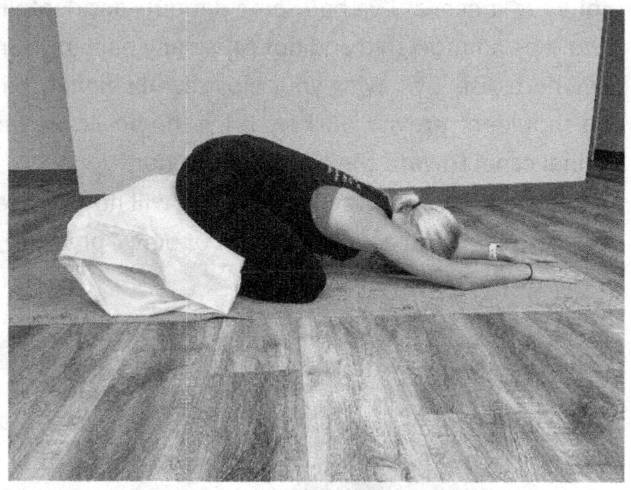

Propping in child's pose position

Bonus thought! Let's say you have a cystocele, you are on a walk with your baby in a stroller, and you feel pelvic pressure. Lean toward the stroller a bit, and this can help the bladder move a bit forward – and often, significantly improve symptoms!

4. **Pelvic floor contractions:** Next, we need to make sure you are supporting the pelvic organs from below by having proper pelvic floor muscle activation throughout your daily activities. Some

patients cannot activate the proper muscles (often, when cued, patient will contract their glutes or abdominals instead) while others can find the right muscles, but strength or endurance are too low for proper pelvic organ support.

Let's pick up some blueberries!

To properly engage your pelvic floor muscles, begin by inhaling through your nose for two seconds while focusing on using your diaphragm and expanding your belly (no chest breathing!). Then, exhale through your mouth and pretend to pick up a blueberry with your vagina. Hold for 1-2 seconds and then release the blueberry all the way back down. Don't rush the let-down part; the relaxation is just as important as the contraction. Repeat for 5 reps, around 4 times a day.

Then, repeat this exercise, but *hold* the blueberry pick-up. Inhale, exhale and pick that blueberry up again. This time, hold it, but don't let your body use "helper" muscles (usually, your glutes, abs, or inner thighs). Some patients begin by holding for 3 seconds, and that is great! If that feels easy to you, hold for 5 seconds or more. The end goal is 10 seconds however most patients take several weeks to work up to that goal. Repeat 5 times, around 4 times a day.

Begin with 20 total pelvic floor muscle contractions daily with half being quick and half being endurance holds. Progress to 40-60 contractions each day.

Listen to your body, and stop if you ever feel any discomfort. Remember, in a pelvic floor physical therapy session, we create a specific exercise program for you so use this as a general guide, modifying based on how your body feels. Does 3 seconds feel too long? No problem, have 2 seconds be your first goal. Is a 5-second hold a piece of cake? Also, great! Try 8 seconds. As always, if *anything* hurts, stop immediately. This should be completely pain-free.

Progress these exercises by then doing them in the seated position and then in standing. Most importantly, start to add them to *real life*.

Remember how we taught you how to blow out on exertion, such as when you lift? Let's add one more thing to support your pelvic organs from below.

To lift: inhale first, exhale and pick up the imaginary blueberry. Now, since you've practiced both exercises separately, you can blow out *and* hold the blueberry while you lift. The blowing out will rid the body of the increased pressure pushing down on your prolapse while the pelvic floor muscle contraction will support the organs from below.

5. **Support garments:** You can also try using specific garments for additional support to help reduce the "falling out tampon" feeling while you are working on improving your pelvic floor muscle strength. Check out the Resources section for some support garments I love!

6. **Pessaries:** Depending on the severity of your prolapse and how much the symptoms interfere with your daily life, some patients will choose to use a pessary. A pessary is a small device (often shaped like a ring or a disc) that is inserted vaginally in order to support the pelvic organs. The pessary must be fitted by a physician however most patients are then able to insert, remove, and clean it on their own. Some patients use a pessary every day for normal life, and other patients may only insert it for high-impact activities, such as running or HIIT training. Pessaries can be a wonderful addition to your action plan however they should not replace the breathing and pelvic floor information provided above.

7. **Collagen:** Supplementing with collagen can help the ligaments that support the pelvic organs. This can be done through foods or collagen supplements/powder. Always check with your physician

before beginning a new supplement. My favorite natural source of collagen through food is bone broth. Some patients like to drink a cup of warm bone broth, and other patients who don't love the taste will cook with it (such as in soups and casseroles).

8. **Sex:** "Will having sex make my prolapse worse?" I hear this all of the time in the clinic. The answer is no. Prolapses are typically soft and simply move out of the way. If sex is uncomfortable due to your prolapse, you can try using gravity to help move the prolapse into a better position. Options to try include laying on your back with a pillow under your hips or on your hands and knees with your forearms dropped down on the bed. If your prolapse is a Grade 4 (past the vaginal opening), you may want to discuss specific options with your physician or a pelvic floor physical therapist.

9. **Surgery:** If conservative treatment has been tried and symptoms of prolapse continue to reach the point where your daily life remains very affected, surgery may be a possibility. Please note that physicians will typically not perform this surgery until you are finished having children. In most all cases, there is not a medical reason why the surgery must be performed; it is chosen when the patient feels the prolapse is severely affecting her quality of life. While knowing surgery may be an option, please know that surgery is usually reserved for more severe cases or ones that have failed conservative management. If you plan to have surgery, it is still essential to properly train your breathing and pelvic floor muscles in order to obtain the most optimal post-op results with the least likelihood of reoccurrence.

Questions

1. Have you ever felt any pelvic pressure or a "falling out" feeling?

2. Place a hand mirror on the floor. Stand over it with your legs apart and separate your labia with your fingers. Do you see any tissue that looks different than before? Often, a prolapse looks like a soft, pink ball.

3. Practice lifting up a box or laundry basket. Did you hold your breath? Now, try again while exhaling and contracting your pelvic floor. How did it feel?

4. Try optimal toileting position for a bowel movement (feet elevated on a stool, forearms on your thighs, and blow out while you gently bear down). How does this compare to how you were doing it before?

Chapter 10:

Feeding Your Baby – However You Do It!

First of all, consider this a judgement-free zone. If you are not pumping or breast feeding, that is completely okay, but your baby is getting fed somehow (likely by you!) so I still want you to read this chapter so you can learn how to do this in the best possible way to avoid hurting yourself.

Ugh, the NICU and feeding. Right?

My twins used feeding tubes for the first three months of our stay before they were allowed to try breast and bottle feeding. I was pumping every three hours like a madwoman. I did...*okay*. My supply was...*okay*. It did the job; I was definitely not an over-producer like some women I know. My twins were so small that in the beginning, they were given only a milliliter or so of breast milk in their feeding tubes so my milk lasted quite a while. They also needed extra calories because of their extremely small size so as the feeds went up, formula was mixed in to increase their caloric intake. This was our particular case and if you have any questions about formula supplementation, please consult your neonatologist, nurse practitioner, or nurse.

So, I pumped...and I pumped....and I pumped. Many of you will know this drill. Because I was exclusively pumping, my husband rented a hospital grade pump for home, and I used a regular pump when I eventually went back to work a few hours a day. I invested in a hands-free pumping bra, and it was probably my favorite purchase throughout all of pregnancy and post-partum. While my twins were in the NICU, I could throw on that pumping bra, pop those cones in, and do whatever I needed to (well, while I was at the table). While it helped my productivity, it also helped my posture since I could sit up straighter and move around a bit so tip #1 is: invest in a hands-free pumping bra.

Three months later, my twins were released to try to nurse as best they could and when I was not there, they would be fed a bottle of breast milk/formula/medication. After a month of this routine, a speech therapist had some suspicions and sure enough, after the swallow study she recommended, we discovered that *both* twins were aspirating breast milk (meaning, it was too thin for them to properly swallow and instead, it was going to their lungs, risking pneumonia). The study continued. The twins were given straight formula; they both still aspirated. From then on, my twins were on formula only (no breast milk) with a thickener, as prescribed by the neonatologist, and my pumping days came to a close. We had a deep freeze full of breast milk that my twins would use when they were older, but for that time period, they could only tolerate the thickened formula without choking and I retired the hands-free bra. So, to be honest, my pumping/breast feeding days were shorter than I had hoped. BUT! I work with post-partum mamas who are breast feeding daily so between their experiences and my training, I can still help out *new* NICU mamas despite my journey not going exactly as I had planned.

I think the most important lesson that comes from my story, though, is that if something happens (as it often does in the NICU) and this affects your breast feeding or pumping, *it is okay.* Once again, I felt guilty because it had been so instilled in me how critical breast milk was for preemies and now, we were no longer giving it to them. Remember, every baby (and every mama) is different, and this is even more apparent in the NICU. Do not worry about what your sister's neighbor's cousin says – chances are, her baby was not even in the NICU and her journey was nothing like yours. Consult with your team – neonatologists, nurses, lactation consultants – and bring up any questions or concerns you have. Remember, you are an important (if not THE most important) person on your baby's care team and whatever you have to say is completely valid. Ask your questions, use your resources, and speak up when you need to. Know that there are many ways for these babies to receive their nutrition, and you have every right to know why any decision is made.

Okay, putting on my physical therapist hat now...let's talk about the mechanics of feeding your baby, either breast feeding or bottle feeding. What do I see often in our clinic? Mamas who are slouching forward to bring their breast to their baby. What can this lead to? Shoulder pain, neck pain, and back pain. Stop for a second and respect how much of your time each day you spend feeding your little one. Let's make it as comfortable as possible.

So much of the time, it's all about the pillows. Use the nursing pillow, use a decorative pillow, use whatever is the most comfortable to you, but the goal is to bring your baby *up to you* as opposed to bringing yourself down to your baby. Ideally, your baby would be safe and supported at a level where he or she can breast or bottle feed while you maintain an upright posture with your shoulder blades relatively down and together.

I also suggest a few stretches for after feeding to open up the chest and stretch the neck.

1. **Upper trap stretch:** Sit up straight with your weight on your sit bones (in other words, no slouching)! The picture demonstrates this stretch sitting on the floor, but you can certainly do it sitting in a chair. Tilt your right ear toward your right shoulder. Place your right hand on top of your head and provide a gentle downward pressure to increase the stretch. Continue to breathe and hold the stretch for 30 seconds. Repeat twice on each side.

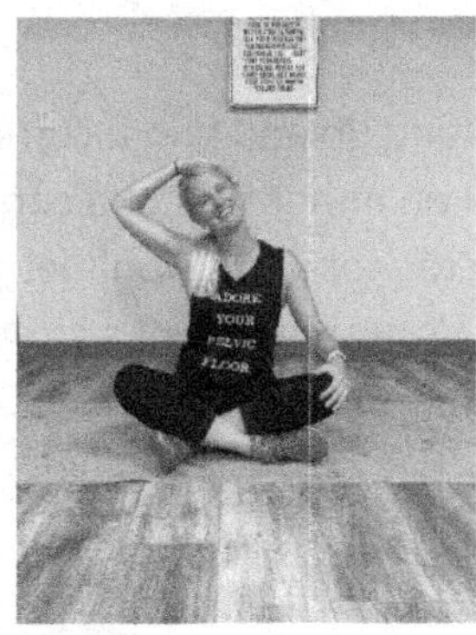

Upper trap stretch

2. **Levator scapulae stretch:** Begin in the same position. This time, while maintaining good posture, angle your head so that your eyes look down into your right armpit. Place your right hand on top and apply gentle pressure to further pull your head toward your right armpit. You should feel the stretch more in the back of the neck this time, as opposed to on the side. Continue to breathe and hold the stretch for 30 seconds. Repeat twice on each side.

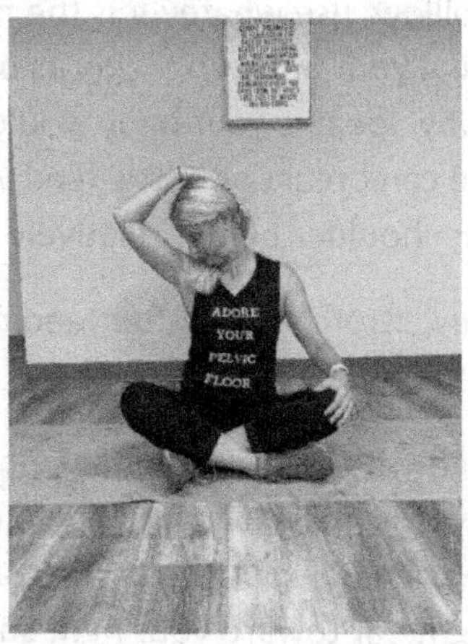

Levator scapulae stretch

3. **Corner stretch:** Stand up and find a corner in your room. Place your hands on the wall on either side of a corner. Place one foot in front of the other and step forward. Don't let your shoulders come up toward your ears! You should feel a stretch across your chest. Continue to breathe while holding for 30 seconds. Repeat twice.

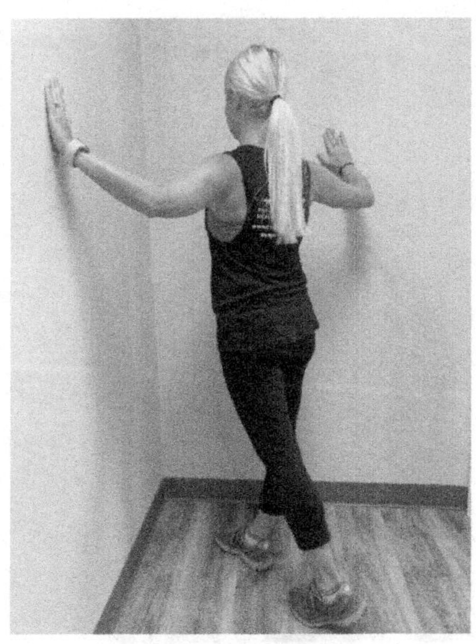

Corner stretch

4. **Self-massage:** Find a firm ball such as a lacrosse ball or baseball. Stand with your back against the wall, placing the ball on the soft tissue between your spine and shoulder blade. Bend your knees and move the ball up and down to find tight muscles and trigger points. When you find a tense area, hold pressure and then move the ball up and down over that area to release tight muscles.

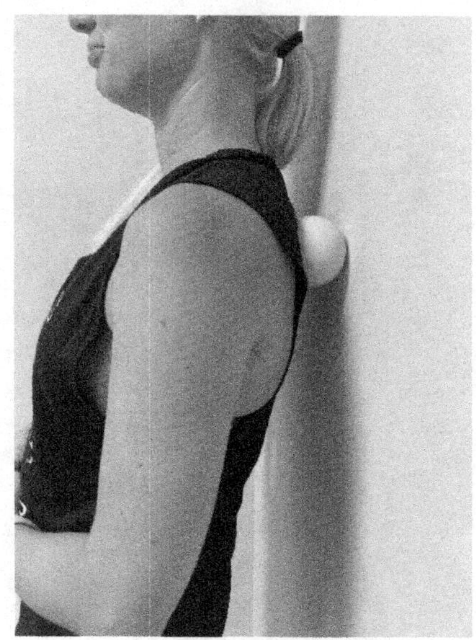

Self-massage

See the Resources section for additional lactation resources. Also, please see Chapters 14 and 15 to address the stress and anxiety that can accompany feeding.

Questions

1. How are you feeding your baby? If your little one is older, how did you feed him or her as a newborn? How did you feel about it?

2. Did feeding come easily to you and your baby? Describe any frustrations. Has anything helped decrease these frustrations?

3. Have you had any shoulder, neck, or upper back pain? Assess your feeding position. Can you improve it by bringing your baby closer to you instead of bringing yourself down to your baby?

4. If you are currently struggling with feeding, what is one step you could take that might make it easier? (Examples: scheduling an appointment with a lactation consultant, buying a hands-free pumping bra, meeting with a support group). Then, take that step!

Chapter 11:
Everybody Poops ... But Do You Do It Right?

In the NICU, pooping is a super big deal. When babies are born prematurely, their bodies have to figure out how to digest days, weeks, or months earlier than planned. The tiniest babies are only fed a couple milliliters at a time, and then they are checked after each feed for any residual feeding that was not digested. Some babies, like my daughter, go days unable to have their first bowel movement despite suppositories and medication. Other babies, often born full-term, have meconium deliveries where they have their first bowel movement prior to delivery and run the risk of aspirating it into their lungs. Nutritionists at the hospital carefully monitor each baby's individual diet plan, checking for nutrients, calories, and fat. As NICU mamas, we often hang on to every bit of this information. How many milliliters did he eat today? Did she digest her entire feeding? Used diapers are checked and recorded.

So...NICU baby poop is super important.

But mamas, your poop is super important, too!

Not everyone's favorite topic, I completely understand. Remember, though, that straining to have a bowel movement can harm your pelvic floor. It can increase your chances of hemorrhoids, pelvic floor muscle dysfunction, and pelvic organ prolapse. Going days between bowel movements can make you feel bloated and have low energy (and mamas, you need that energy!). Plus, remember, a large portion of your immunity comes from your gut so if there was ever a time to reassess your gut health, now is the time.

What is "normal" for bowel movements? The technical definition says bowel movements should be in a range from three times a day up to every three days without the need for straining. I have to add, please realize that everyone is different. Many people would feel absolutely terrible if they didn't have a bowel movement for three days. I tell my patients a good goal is to have a bowel movement at least once every 1-2 days without straining, and more is okay as long as the stool is normal (formed, but soft).

Many women become constipated during pregnancy (thanks, hormones), and this can continue into the post-partum period, especially in times of stress and variable schedules (hello, NICU). So, what can you do if you are struggling to have a comfortable, daily bowel movement?

1. **Hydrate:** Many people in general struggle to consume enough water each day, and it's even harder if water bottles are not allowed in your little one's room. The problem with too little water is that you develop hard stool – sometimes small pellets – and these are uncomfortable to pass. Aim to drink enough water that when you urinate, the urine is a light straw color. You can also take your body weight and divide it by two to give you a general guideline of the number of ounces to take in each day (so if you weigh 200 pounds, your goal might be 100 ounces of water). Drink water on your way to the NICU, drink water in the parent lounge, and drink on your way home. Hydration is also critical for nursing and pumping mamas so while you increase your water intake to improve the consistency of your stool, it should help you produce milk for your little one as well!

2. **Toileting position:** If you have an older toddler, observe them as they poop into their diaper. What is their go-to position? They squat down, right? That is because their body is naturally guiding them to the best position to have a bowel movement. Unfortunately, this is not the position we use on our westernized toilets. So, what can we do?

   Use one of my favorite pelvic floor products out there – a Squatty Potty!

The Squatty Potty is a wide step stool that is about 7-9 inches tall (they have different ones to choose from) that sits beneath you when you are seated on your toilet to have a bowel movement. By placing your feet up onto the stool, it helps your pelvic floor relax, and it also improves the path your poop has to travel, essentially eliminating going around a corner. For best results, place your feet up on the Squatty Potty, lean forward so your forearms are resting on your thighs, and blow out through your mouth as if you were blowing out birthday candles. Blowing out, like we have discussed before, rids the body of increased air pressure, protecting the pelvic floor.

If you already have another step stool at home, feel free to try it out first before purchasing something new. I have plenty of patients who use something they already have or have made with milk crates or other items, but be aware that the benefit of the Squatty Potty is that it has a cutout so you can push it back against the toilet and out of the way so it decreases your chances of tripping over a stool in the middle of the night.

What do you do when you are not at home (like in the NICU bathroom)? If it's a single stall and the trash can is fairly empty, you can always turn it sideways and place your feet up on the trash can. If that isn't possible in your restroom, at the very least, lean forward with your forearms on your thighs and blow out when you gently bear down.

3. **Abdominal bowel massage:** When you eat your food, it travels down your esophagus into your stomach, into your small intestines, then into your large intestines (often called the colon) before finally moving into the rectum and then out of your body. When patients come into the clinic and mention they only have a bowel movement every 4-5 days – or even once a week – the first technique I often recommend is abdominal bowel massage. The large intestines travel up your right side, across your abdomen, down your left side, and then it curves a little before it connects to your rectum. By

performing abdominal bowel massage, a patient is not physically pushing the stool through but instead, stimulating the muscles of the large intestine to contract and move stool along its pathway.

- Begin lying down or reclining back.
- Lift up your shirt and gently take two fingers and place them on the lower right side of your abdomen (think of it as in line with your nipple but down above your pelvis).
- Massage gentle circles traveling from the lower right part of the abdomen to the upper right part of the abdomen until you reach just beneath your ribs.
- When you reach the level of your ribs, stop moving upward and instead, continue to massage circles, this time moving across your upper abdomen toward the left.
- Once you reach the left side (again, about even with the nipple), keep massaging but move downward to the lower left part of the abdomen.
- Once you reach the bottom, pick up your hand and place it on the bottom right part of the abdomen, beginning again.
- Do this for 5 minutes, twice each day, if you are struggling with constipation and/or slow motility.

4. **Increase natural fiber while decreasing processed foods:** Assess your diet. Work on increasing your consumption of whole grains, leafy greens, berries, and lean protein while decreasing processed foods. Try mixing flax or chia seeds into smoothies or oatmeal.

5. **Probiotics:** Probiotics are an excellent addition to your diet in order to promote optimal bowel health, especially during times of stress. You can get probiotics by consuming foods such as kombucha tea, fermented foods, and certain yogurts. In addition, probiotics are available in supplement and powder form. Talk to your doctor about which option might be right for you. In general, probiotics with multiple strains of lactobacillus are a great option as this

increases the good bacteria that are naturally present in your gut and vaginal region (note – these probiotics are often refrigerated).

6. **Warm fluid in the morning:** Many people notice that bowel movements are often stimulated after a warm cup of coffee in the morning. A little coffee is fine, but if you are having any urinary symptoms (such as leakage or urinary frequency), you will want to limit this as coffee is a bladder irritant and will likely make these symptoms worse. If you are not a coffee drinker, or if you need to avoid it for bladder reasons, you can start your day with a simple warm cup of water. While it might not be the tastiest, the warmth will help stimulate your bowels, increasing your chances of starting your day with a good bowel movement.

7. **Getting up earlier than you need to:** If you are in a rush when you first get up (such as hurrying to the NICU or rushing to a shift at work prior to visiting your baby), your body does not have enough time to "rest and digest" in order to stimulate a good bowel movement. I understand you are most likely exhausted, however on the days when you feel like you can tolerate it, try to get up fifteen minutes earlier. This will give you a chance to actually sit down and eat some breakfast while consuming some warm liquid and maybe performing some abdominal bowel massage, all in order to stimulate a bowel movement before you begin the craziness that may become your day.

Questions

1. How often do you have a bowel movement? Do you usually have to strain?

2. How does your abdominal region feel? Do you feel bloated? Do you have gas?

3. If you are struggling with constipation, what is one change you are willing to make in order to improve your bowel movements?

Chapter 12:

Bridge the Gap: Treating a Diastasis

First of all, let's all remember that no one's abdominal region looks strong and recovered immediately post-partum. As a society, we are fed images of celebrities on the beach a few weeks post-partum with flat stomachs and six-packs (shout out to the celebrities who have shared real photos in order to educate women on what the post-partum period actually looks like). Also, that story you heard about your sister's best friend's neighbor who was back to CrossFit a month post-partum? Not the normal (and also, not recommended – see Chapter 16 on returning to exercise). That being said, maybe you are a few weeks (or years) post-partum and when looking in a full-length mirror at your belly, something just doesn't look *right*. Maybe you still look four months pregnant. Maybe you notice what appears to be a gap in the middle of your belly. Maybe if you touch above your belly button, it feels like you can push your finger deeper into your abdomen than you suspect is normal.

You may have what is called a diastasis rectus abdominus, or DRA for short. A diastasis is a gapping at the linea alba – a line of connective tissue that runs vertically down the center of your rectus abdominus ("six-pack" muscles). It may surprise you to learn that *most* women experience this condition by the end of pregnancy, and whether or not you have a large DRA is largely determined by your genetics (thanks, Mom). This separation can be measured by ultrasound or by a manual assessment. Manual assessments are best performed by a trained physical therapist however you can attempt to assess yourself using your own hand or a partner's.

Lay on your bed with your knees bent. Place two fingers right above your belly button, and push down gently. Lift your head up off the table. You are feeling for a gap between the two sides of the rectus muscle; officially, a separation of more than two finger widths is considered a DRA. Recent literature has found that even more important that the width of the separation is the depth – do you feel like you can push your fingers deep down into your abdomen? Complete this check directly above and below the belly button as well as four inches above and below the belly button. Another issue to watch for with a DRA is referred to as coning. Often seen when trying to sit directly up, look down or have a partner assess to see if an area along your midline pushes outward. Lastly, place an open hand across your abdomen. Contract your abdominals and assess what you feel. Do you feel activation of the muscles? Do you feel equal contraction among lower, middle, and upper abdominals? (Spoiler alert – often, it's the lower abdominals that activate the least and need to be addressed).

Okay, so let's say you think you notice a diastasis. Or, let's say you don't, but you do notice that your abdominals don't seem to be contracting properly. First of all, remain calm. This (and prolapse) seem to be the diagnoses where patients come in basically freaking out. Use this concern to your favor to keep you from doing something you shouldn't be doing yet (running, squats, worrying about immediately losing all of that baby weight). Remember, as previously mentioned with other pelvic floor dysfunctions, this is common but not normal. Again, many women have a DRA post-partum; what is important is that you take steps to properly rehab it. And YES, once again, you can do this while sitting right next to your baby's isolette.

1. **Postural awareness (review from Chapter 1):** Many post-partum women stand in one of two positions – either with a forward tilted pelvis and a large sway in the low back OR standing with their hips pushed forward, clenching their glutes. Neither allows the abdominals to activate the way they need to in order to do their job. Check out your posture from the side using either a large mirror or a timed full body selfie. Place one hand at your bra line and one at the level of your waistband. If you are standing with a large sway in your back, I want you to shift your pelvis (tuck your tailbone) so that your two hands come closer together. Now, instead of elongated abdominals that cannot contract, you have brought them into the correct

position so that they can function. If you are standing with your pelvis pushed forward, try to bring your hips back directly beneath your rib cage so that your glutes can unclench and you can engage those abs.

2. **Abdominal awareness and the "Zip-it-up" exercise:** Now that you are in the correct posture, you want to contract the proper region of the abdominals. Most people are more dominant in the upper and middle abdominals, with less activation and strength in the lower abdominals. This is even more common in pregnant and post-partum women. To correct this, imagine you have a zipper that runs vertically from your pubic bone to your belly button. To properly contract the lower abdominals, inhale first through your nose using your diaphragm (your belly should expand). Then, exhale through your mouth and "zip" the lower abdominals up from the pubic bone to the belly button. This is not a large contraction; think of it more as an activation. Hold this for 5 seconds and then relax. Do this 10 times, twice each day.

3. **"Blow as you go" (aka your new BFF):** Imagine you are trying to help a friend pick up a really heavy couch. What do we do? We grab a hold of it, suck in our breath and try to pick it up. Now imagine you have weakness and a gap in the front of your abdomen, such as with a diastasis. When you hold your breath, where will all of that air go? Quick answer – it will find the point of least resistance (in other words, your most vulnerable point), and it will go there. If you hold your breath during exertion, all of that air pressure will push directly out on the weak area of your abdomen (or to a weak area of your pelvic floor, if you have that as well). Not the greatest result. So, to prevent this air pressure pressing on your belly, I want you to work on what is called "exhale on exertion," or, as many patients prefer, "blow

as you go." Let's say you are going to stand up out of a chair. Inhale first, exhale and zip the lower abdominals. Then, continue to blow out and zip WHILE you stand up. Same thing goes for lifting a bag. Inhale first, exhale and zip. Then, blow out and continue to zip WHILE you lift. Fast forward to a week or six months, whenever your little one comes home. You need to pick up the carseat. Inhale first, exhale and zip. Continue to blow out and zip WHILE you lift the carseat. You will forget a lot in the beginning and that is completely normal. The goal is that the more you do this during your normal daily activities, the more it will become automatic. Down the road, you may go to contract your abdominals and realize that they have already assumed the correct position.

4. **Kinesiotape:** Kinesiotape is a stretchy, cotton-based tape that can be used for many different purposes. With my patients who have a diastasis, I love to use kinesiotape to better approximate the abdominals (in other words, "close the gap" by bringing the abdominal muscles closer together) so that the muscles can relearn how to activate in the proper position. To perform this technique, cut six pieces of kinesiotape, each three blocks. Begin by placing one piece below the sternum. Anchor the tail, then gently pull the tape down and in the opposite direction. Stick the other end to your skin, without pulling the end of the tape. Do the same thing on the other side, making an "X." Make a second "X," right above the belly button. Do once again, right below the belly button. Each piece of tape should pull gently toward the midline, bringing the abdominals together. As always, consult a physical therapist if you have difficulty with this technique.

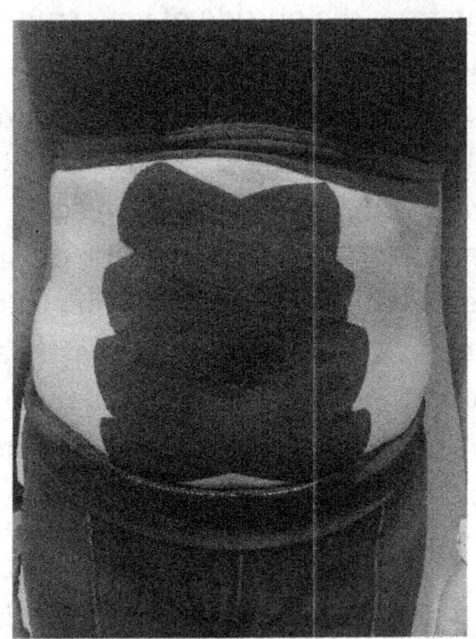

Kinesiotape for DRA

5. **Avoiding coning:** This one is somewhat controversial. Some physical therapists are okay with their patients completing exercises that cause a little bit of coning at the midline; I still prefer to adjust the activity so that coning does not occur. If you notice yourself completing any activity that leads to coning at your midline, try to engage your abdominals by zipping from the bottom to the top. If the coning still occurs, try a different exercise instead. When getting up out of bed, many mamas have coning if they sit straight up. A better choice would be to first roll onto your side, breathe in, then exhale and engage your abdominals as you use your arms to push yourself up to the seated position.

6. **Abdominal muscle soft tissue work:** Sometimes mamas have tightness in their obliques (ab muscles on the sides) which can promote a DRA staying apart by pulling the rectus muscles to the outside. Take your thumb (and a little coconut oil if you

prefer) and place it on the side of your abdominals. Gently drag your thumb from the outside of your trunk in toward your midline. Notice if any tissue feels firm or restricted. Massage the same area again from the outside in. Move your thumb down a little and repeat. Do this from right beneath your ribs down toward your hip then perform again on the other side. Remember, always massage from the outside in to bring the tissue together. If you feel an area that is tight (less soft than the other areas), give it a little bit of extra attention. For NICU mamas still in the NICU, this can be done in your baby's room while sitting or standing, just slip your thumb right underneath your shirt!

For further progression of exercises you can use to improve a diastasis, please refer to Chapter 16. If possible, especially if you know you have a diastasis, please see a qualified physical therapist for proper diagnosis and an individualized treatment plan.

Questions

1. If you think you might have a DRA, lay down and complete the self-assessment. Can you feel a gap between the rectus muscles? Do you notice coning or increased depth? Are you able to engage your muscles across the gap?

2. Check your posture. Are your ribs and pelvis in line or is one in front of the other? Are you able to correct this? How does it feel?

3. Pick up a box or laundry backet. What is your breathing pattern? Do you hold your breath? If so, try lifting it again while blowing out and engaging your abs. How does it feel now?

Chapter 13:

NICU Baby and Chill: Post-Partum Sex

Six weeks after your delivery, you follow-up with your OB-GYN, and she gives you the full release – you can return to sex, running, boot camp classes, ultra-marathons, and hiking Mt. Kilimanjaro (pelvic floor physical therapists everywhere drop their heads in disgust). We've talked about how ridiculous the six-week "release to everything" concept is already, but let's focus here on what it means for sex.

First of all, if you (or your partner) think that women everywhere get this release and immediately go home to have lovely, lingering sexual experiences without pain while their baby sleeps peacefully, please remove this "ideal" from your brain. I'm sure there are some women out there who fall into this category, but after treating post-partum women for over thirteen years, let me assure you that this is not the majority of women. First of all, do not feel pressure to jump right back into the bedroom once you hit six-weeks post-partum (this goes for any mama, not just NICU mamas). Whether you have a baby at home or a baby in the NICU, chances are you are overwhelmed and sleep deprived which doesn't typically leave you excited to grab your partner and run to the bed. If you do feel comfortable and ready to give it a go, that's wonderful and I don't want to discourage you at all. I simply want to ensure that any woman who doesn't feel ready should never feel pressured or that she is the only one out there delaying the return to sex, because I promise you that this is completely normal. Add having a baby in the NICU on top of everything else, and this may be the furthest thing from your mind and *that is okay.* You will know when you are ready.

If you are at the point right now when you are not ready, please still read through this chapter. There are many techniques you can start doing now which help make the transition to intercourse easier whenever you do feel ready whether that is in one month or ten. If you have returned to sex and aren't having problems, then that's great! As a pelvic floor physical therapist, though, I work every day with women who struggle to return to intercourse so I want to make sure I get as much information as I can out there to our NICU mamas who may need to hear this.

To get the first myth out of the way, you can still have discomfort in the vaginal region even if you had a c-section. It is true that you didn't deliver your baby vaginally, but remember that you were also pregnant – whether that was for a full 40 weeks or six months, like me. No matter what, your body went through major changes and increased pressure was placed on your pelvic floor. Some c-sections are planned and others are performed after a mama has pushed for a while so there was still a "pushing" element involved. Even if the c-section occurred without pushing (again, me), the surgeons cut through seven layers of tissue in your abdomen to remove your baby. That means that you have healing tissue not just at your c-section scar, but deep into your abdomen which is a close neighbor to your pelvic floor. In addition, your abdominal muscles are separated during a c-section to reach the uterus so there is a great deal of weakness here after surgery and when the lower abdominals aren't activating properly, other muscles try to jump in and help. A common group wanting to help? That's right, the pelvic floor. This can lead to an overactive pelvic floor which means that these muscles are too tense, gripping when they shouldn't be, and this can lead to pain with sex.

Review of pelvic anatomy

Remember, the pelvic floor is made up of fourteen different muscles that begin around your pubic bone in the front, go underneath you like a sling or hammock, and attach around your tailbone in the back. These are super important muscles that are responsible for:

1. Keeping you continent (bladder and bowel)
2. Supporting your pelvic organs (bladder, uterus, rectum)
3. Sexual function (an orgasm is actually many, very fast contractions of the pelvic floor)
4. Core stabilization

So, what's going on with painful sex post-partum? (Side note – you could have even had this before pregnancy; we see people for painful sex all the time who have never been pregnant). Often, the pelvic floor muscles are too tense – think of them like gripping, clenching, or holding their breath. These muscles should experience a natural lengthening every time you inhale and for many of my patients with pelvic floor pain, this isn't happening – the muscles are a bit "stuck." Then, if you can imagine penetration (so yes, sex, but this could also be something like a speculum, tampon, or menstrual cup when your period returns), it's a sudden stretch to a tight muscle group. Imagine a runner who has tight hamstrings and suddenly you forcefully stretch her straight leg up toward her head. Ouch.

Another way I describe this to patients is to think about when you've been sitting at a computer or leaning over a project for a long time. Have you ever noticed tension that becomes present in your neck or have you noticed your shoulders creeping up toward your ears? That's tension in your shoulder and neck muscles, and that is a very good comparison to what is happening in your pelvic floor. You aren't telling your muscles to grip and you may not even be aware that they are, but once you know what to watch for, you can work on properly letting them go.

In addition to muscle tightness, you can also have scar tissue and sensitivity that can be from a tear during vaginal delivery, an episiotomy, or around your c-section scar. Adhesions can clamp tissue down and keep it from gliding and sliding like it should. This (along with the muscle tension that may also be present) restricts blood flow and can restrict the nerves that innervate the area, leading to pain and dysfunction. Nerves can become extra sensitive perceiving simple touch as severe pain.

Another concern I have heard from NICU mamas specifically is fear of sex because they are afraid of becoming pregnant again. I was the same way. It took my husband and I four years, four IVF cycles, and an egg donor to become pregnant...but at that six-week follow-up while my twins were still on ventilators, I requested birth control because I was deathly afraid of some type of medical miracle that would leave me pregnant. I can certainly understand this fear during such an overwhelming time. You can talk to your doctor about options, and you can also *wait if you don't feel ready*. I want you to be able to return to pain-free sex when you are ready, but I also don't want you to feel any pressure toward intimacy if it is not right for you at this time.

Let's say you are interested in returning to intimacy, but you're either not sure where to start or you've tried, but it hurt. What should you do?

Plan for returning to sex after baby – either BEFORE you have attempted OR if you have attempted and have had pain

1. **Begin with my favorite exercise, diaphragmatic breathing:** Remember, this is also the awesome exercise that is going to help everything from your bowel and bladder function to stabilizing your baby's oxygen saturation and heart rate during kangaroo care. Breathe in deeply through your nose for at least two seconds, focusing on expanding your abdomen and letting your ribs raise up and out. Then exhale out through your mouth for two to four seconds, letting the abdomen and ribs return back to neutral. *THIS NEXT PART IS NEW!* When you inhale using your diaphragm, your diaphragm should naturally move downward and so should the pelvic floor which is what we need it to do – lengthen and relax. When you are working on this breathing technique, begin by imagining your "sit bones" separating and your pelvic floor lengthening every time you inhale and then imagine them returning to neutral every time you exhale. After practice, focus on these muscles and you should start to feel a gentle downward movement of these muscles when you breathe in. Start doing this as much you can now (remember, you can do this during kangaroo care!) and when you are ready for sex, do this before, during, and afterward to help the muscles relax.

2. **LUBE:** This is important for several reasons. First of all, you're returning to sex after delivering a baby so let's pull out all the stops to make this as easy as possible. You have less estrogen being produced during pregnancy and while breast feeding (these hormonal changes will be present until about three months after the very last time you nurse/pump OR three months after delivery if you choose not to breast feed). Less estrogen means thinner and more sensitive vaginal tissue as well as decreased lubrication. Beware of some common lubricants that are highly marketed as they can contain chemicals that cause irritation and may even lead to vaginal tissue damage. See the Resources section at the back of the book for my favorites!

3. **Stretches**: The following are stretches I love to help promote pelvic floor muscle relaxation.

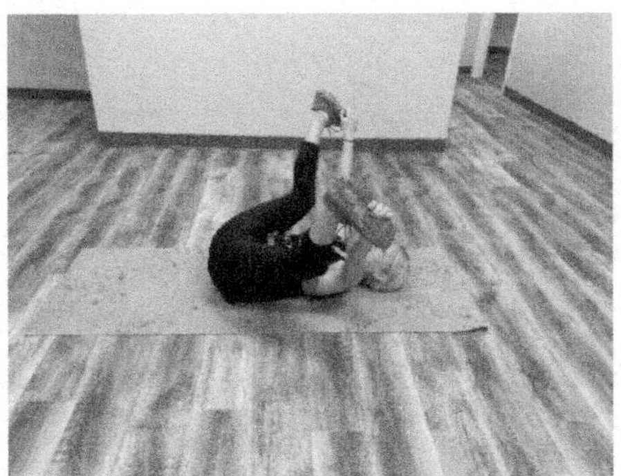

Happy baby stretch

Happy baby: Lay on your back with your knees bent and your hands grasping the inside of your arches. Inhale and focus on lengthening the pelvic floor, imagining your sit bones separating. Exhale and let your pelvic floor return to neutral. Hold for 5 deep breaths. Repeat twice.

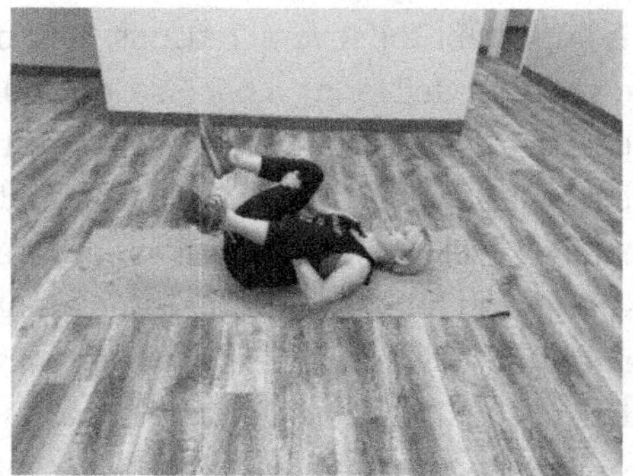

Modified happy baby stretch

Modified happy baby: Lay on your back with your knees bent and apart, holding with your hands beneath your knees. Inhale and focus on relaxing the pelvic floor, imagining your sit bones separating. Exhale and let your pelvic floor return to neutral. Hold for 5 deep breaths. Repeat twice.

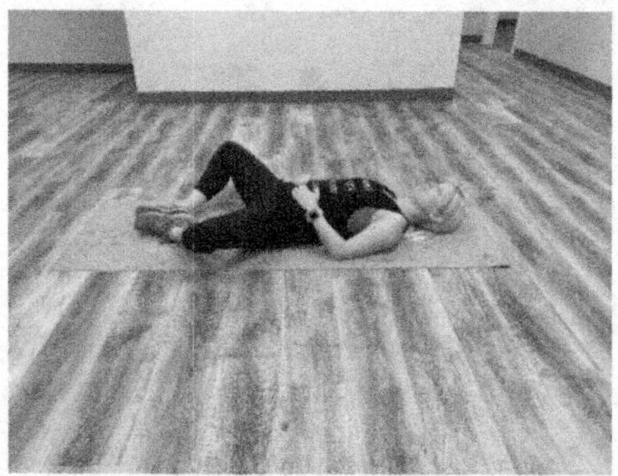

Butterfly stretch

Butterfly stretch: Lay on your back and let your knees fall to either side. If this is uncomfortable, move your feet down further away from your trunk or add pillows beneath your knees. Inhale and focus on lengthening the pelvic floor. Exhale and let your pelvic floor return to neutral. Hold for 5 deep breaths. Repeat twice

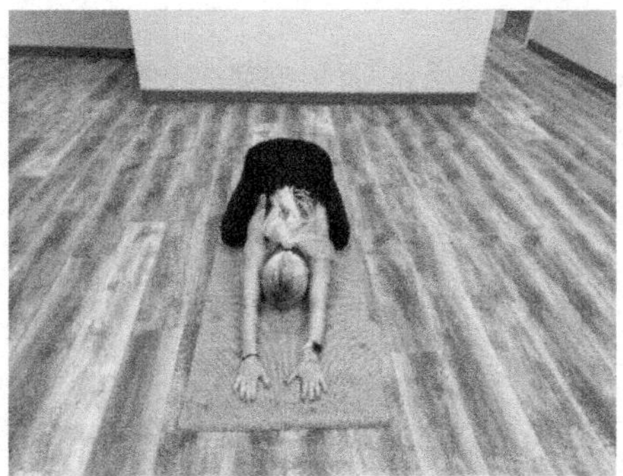

Child's pose

Child's pose: Begin on your hands and knees with your feet together and your knees apart. Sit back, moving your hips toward your heels (they might touch or they might not, and either is fine). Reach your arms forward and tuck your head to relax. Inhale and focus on lengthening the pelvic floor, imagining your sit bones separating. Exhale and let your pelvic floor return to neutral. Hold for 5 deep breaths or longer.

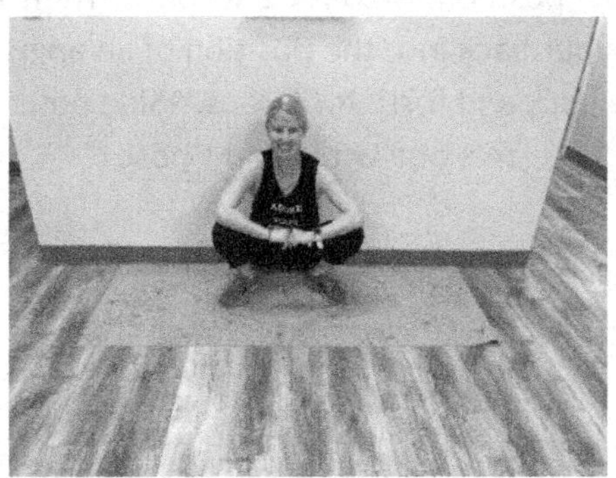

Deep squat

Deep squat: Drop into a full squat with your back against a walk or your hand holding something for balance. If your heels cannot touch the ground, place a small, rolled-up towel under each heel. Fully relax your pelvic floor. Complete at least 5 deep, diaphragmatic breaths or longer if it feels good. Proceed carefully with this one if you have a more severe prolapse.

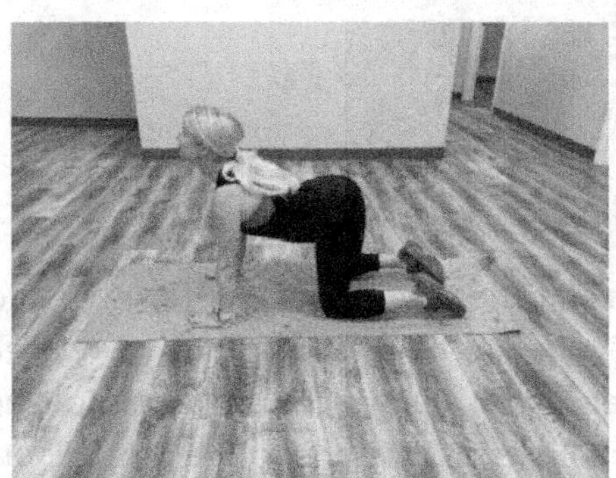 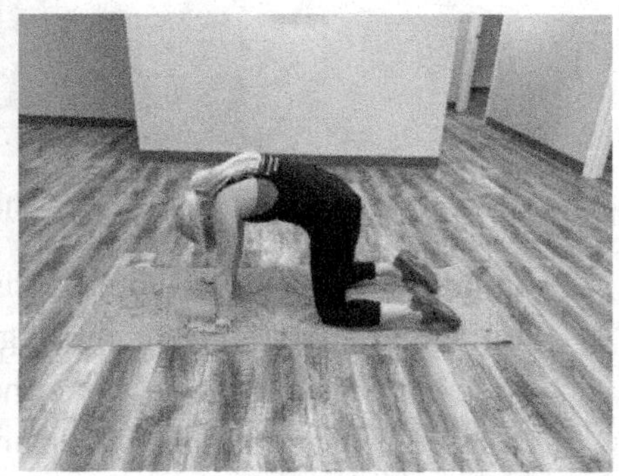

Cat/cow

Cat/cow: Begin on your hands and knees. Inhale, look up, and sway your back into the "cow" position. Hold for 2 seconds. Then, exhale, tuck your head, and arch your back into the position of an angry cat. Hold for 2 seconds. Alternate back and forth for 5 reps. *Side note: I love to alternate this one with child's pose!

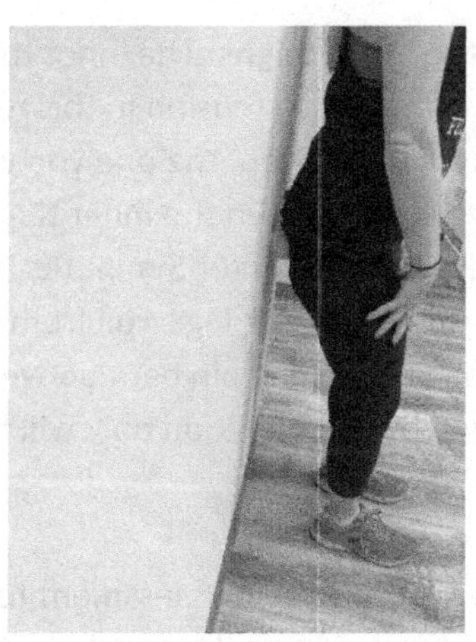

Soft tissue massage to hips

Soft tissue massage to the back of the hips: The hip muscles are the next-door neighbors of the pelvic floor. During and after pregnancy, the muscles in the back of the hips are often very tight (thanks to pregnancy hormones, see Chapter 1). To help reduce the tension, place a lacrosse ball on the soft tissue on the back of your hip and back up against a wall. Massage the back of both hips for 5 minutes total.

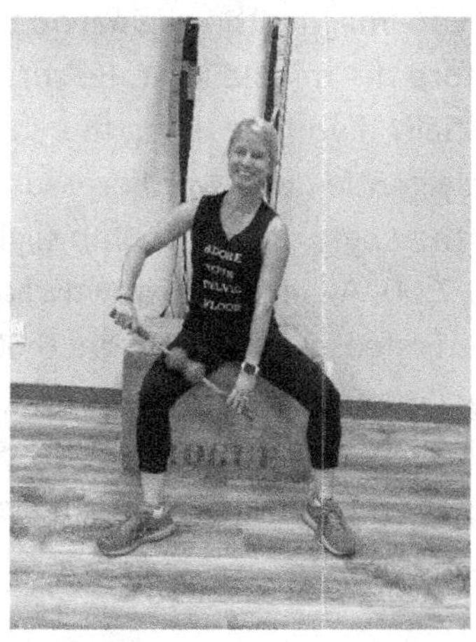

Soft tissue massage to inner thighs

Soft tissue massage to the inner thighs: The inner thigh muscles attach up in the pelvis and many women have tension in this region that can affect the pelvic floor. Take a rolling pin (yep, the one you would use to make pie or cookies!) and massage up and down the inner thighs, focusing on any area that feels tight. Roll comfortably for 5 minutes. If you are recently post-partum or have swelling in your lower legs, roll from right above the knee up your leg and then place the rolling pin back above the knee again. Focusing on rolling in the upward direction only will help reduce swelling.

4. **Thumb stretch:** This can be an assessment tool for you if you want to check to see how your muscles are doing PRIOR to attempting sex and also a treatment if there is tension. Do not do if this causes pain, and you should always see a pelvic floor physical therapist if you are struggling. Also, wait until after your six-week follow-up appointment before you assess. You can complete this self-stretch either laying on your back with some pillows propped behind your back or (often easier) standing up in the shower with one foot propped up on the edge of the bathtub, stool, or whatever else you have. Make sure the nail on your thumb is trimmed. Then, gently insert your thumb, pad-side down, into the bottom of the vaginal opening (6:00 if you imagine the vaginal opening as a clock) to the depth of just before the middle joint. Be sure to use lubricant (see Resources) especially if you are doing this somewhere other than the shower. Apply gentle downward pressure for 30 seconds, then release. Change the angle of your thumb slightly as if you were going to press at 7:00. Again, press downward gently for 30 seconds, and then release. Perform from 6:00 to 10:00 and then 6:00 to 2:00 (if you are standing up in the shower, you'll have to stop and switch which foot is up depending on which side you are treating). Do this for 3-5 minutes, every 1-2 days, if you are having tension or pain.

5. **Pelvic wands:** Sometimes it's too awkward to work on your pelvic floor with just your thumb or sometimes the muscles that are tense are deeper than you can reach. In these cases, I recommend one of my very favorite pelvic health tools – a pelvic wand. Pelvic wands are "S" shaped wands that can be made of different materials, but my favorite is one made from silicone as it is much more comfortable. Similar to the thumb stretch, you can use a pelvic wand lying in bed with your back propped up, in the shower, or in any other position you find comfortable. Apply lubricant (but not a silicone-based lubricant on a silicone wand as it can break down the material), and insert the wand at the bottom opening of the vagina (again, 6:00). A very slight insertion will reach the muscles closest to the opening while insertion to the first curve of the wand will reach the deep muscles. By moving the handle to the side, gently stretch the tissue from 6:00 to 8:00. Perform this a few times, feeling free to hold pressure anywhere that you feel you need to work on more. Then, gently stretch from 8:00 to 10:00. When you have finished this side, complete the same technique on the other side. You can stretch with a pelvic wand for up to 10 minutes, every 1-2 days as needed. There is also a vibrating wand which is especially nice for mamas having pain in the pelvic floor. By inserting the wand and holding the vibrating end on a tight/tender location, it brings increased blood flow to the area, encouraging the muscle to let go (though you wouldn't want to use this one in the shower). Another option is a pelvic wand that can be warmed in a cup of hot water or cooled in the freezer. When patients feel ready to return to sex, some prefer to stretch with the pelvic wand for a few minutes as a "warm-up" prior to sexual intimacy. Please see the Resources section for pelvic wand recommendations and a discount code. BONUS: If and when you decide to become pregnant again, you can use this same wand toward the end of pregnancy to complete perineal massage in order to stretch the tissue and prepare for a vaginal delivery or VBAC, if that is what you choose.

6. **Dilators:** When patients come in with extreme apprehension about returning to intercourse or if a single-finger exam is extremely painful, I may recommend the use of vaginal dilators instead of a pelvic wand. The difference is that a pelvic wand is one size with an S-shaped curve while dilators are straight with a curved tip and come in a range of sizes. The idea with dilator use is that instead of going straight from no insertion to full penetration, you can work on your own by starting with inserting a small size dilator and over time, working up to the larger sizes. These can help all mamas in terms of muscle stretching however I think a huge additional benefit is that they tend to give women more confidence in returning to intercourse and typically help lessen the sudden tensing of the pelvic floor many women experience when they are nervous to have any type of penetration. Think of it like returning to walking or elliptical after a knee injury prior to running, with the added benefit of muscle stretch. When patients feel ready to return to sex, some prefer to stretch with a dilator for a few minutes as a "warm-up" prior to sexual intimacy. See the Resources section for dilator recommendations and a discount code.

7. **Positions:** When returning to sex, some positions may be more comfortable than others, and I strongly urge you to change positions any time you feel pain. Every patient is different however over the years working with women who have pain with sex, certain positions tend to lead to a bit more success. One position that may be good to try is having the female partner on top as this allows her to control the depth and speed of penetration, making her feel more in control with less anxiety. Another option that promotes pelvic floor muscle relaxation is having the female partner being on hands and knees, possibly dropping down onto her forearms into a modified child's pose (also, this can be very helpful if you have a prolapse). Another great option for prolapse can be the female partner laying on her back with a pillow under her hips so that gravity can move the pelvic organs back to their ideal position

during that time. Every mama is different; these positions may not work for you at all. Experiment with this, and try to find what feels best to you.

8. **Read through the next two chapters!** Having a little one in the NICU (even if they have "graduated" and gone home) can be very traumatic. Our mental health is closely related to our nervous system, and if our nervous system is constantly in "fight, flight, or freeze," it makes tissues more sensitive and can increase muscle tension. Do your best to address your mental health so that you may obtain your best physical healing.

9. **Still having trouble?** Find a pelvic health physical therapist! See the Resources section in the back of the book to find one in your area.

Questions

1. Where are you on your journey of returning to intimacy? How does this make you feel (nervous, excited, overwhelmed, etc.)?

2. How did you imagine you would return to intimacy after having a baby? How has this compared to real life?

3. If you have returned to sex, did you have pain? How did you feel emotionally?

4. Are you able to talk about this with your partner?

5. Turn on some calm music and try the yoga stretches, focusing on breathing and lengthening your pelvic floor. Compare how you feel before and afterward.

6. If you are having pain, how do you feel about trying a pelvic wand or dilators? Which do you feel would best help you (feel free to look at the website listed in the Resources section to check them out before you answer)?

7. Try the self-assessment with the thumb stretch (if you are 6 weeks or more post-partum). Did you feel tenderness and if so, where (ex: 6:00, 8:00, etc.)? Record where you feel tenderness and how strong the discomfort is on a 0-10 scale. You can use this to compare to how you feel in the future after working on the thumb stretch for a few weeks.

Chapter 14:
Running From Tigers: The Mind-Body Connection

NICU brain.

I may have made up the term, but ladies – this is a real, physiological process that is happening in your brain during the time of your NICU stay (and can extend to when you come home so don't skip to the next chapter, mamas that are at home). Hang with me as I tell you how the NICU is similar to a tiger.

Our brains are hard-wired to protect us and save our lives. So, let's say you are walking down the street and out of nowhere, a tiger appears and begins sprinting toward you, teeth bared. This immediately triggers your body's alarm system. An almond-shaped structure in your brain called the amygdala sends a signal to your hypothalamus which then signals your pituitary gland to tell your adrenal glands to release your stress hormones, cortisol and epinephrine. This leads to what you may have heard of – the "fight, flight, or freeze" response. Back up from the tiger for a moment and think about a time you had to give a presentation in front of your class or coworkers. What did you feel? Butterflies in your stomach, your heart racing, your palms sweating. These were actual physiological processes that occurred because your brain was trying to save you from the impending tiger attack (or in that moment, public speaking). When faced with an attack, your body is going to instantly make multiple changes that are going to make you better able to run away or fight. Your pupils dilate so you can see better. Your heart rate and blood pressure increase. Blood shifts away from organ systems that aren't necessary in the moment, such as your gut and your reproductive system, and TOWARD areas like your arms and legs that you will need to fight or race away. You become on edge because you *need* to be – you need full attention to be able to know what the tiger is doing and to be aware enough to know how to get away from it. You have a temporarily decreased ability to learn and can have difficulty with your memory because in that moment, those brain functions are not needed to save your life. You may not feel pain in the same way you normally would. If you twist your ankle while running from the tiger, your brain weighs which is more dangerous – the sprinting tiger or a twisted ankle. The tiger will win and you'll be able to run away without feeling your ankle (until later, when you are safe and then the pain will begin).

Are you recognizing some of the symptoms you might be feeling in the NICU?

Here is an example of the power of the mind-body connection. My twins were born via emergency c-section at 11:40 and 11:42 in the morning. Following protocol, the nurse got me up to sit at the edge of my hospital bed exactly twelve hours later to try to pump. It was excruciating; with every movement, it felt like daggers piercing my abdomen, and I had to rely on the nurse to basically sit me up because I was unable to move on my own. We tried a bit of pumping – no luck – and then she had to help me lay back down. I felt like I'd run a marathon.

The crazy part came an hour and a half later.

One of the NICU nurse practitioners came downstairs to give me an update. Hannah was somewhat stable, but Gavin was "having a rough night." They had moved him to an oscillator (a more powerful ventilator) and had given him several surfactant treatments to help his breathing. He had stabilized a bit, but it was touch and go. I thanked her for the information and while I was laying there, feeling stranded while my babies were fighting for their lives a floor above me, my nurse came in and said it would be okay if she took me upstairs in the wheelchair. This hadn't been an option up to this point, and mamas, when I said yes, she started to walk toward me, and *I got out of the bed and walked over to the wheelchair.* An hour and a half earlier, I could not sit up without help and this time, I stood up, walked over to the wheelchair, and sat down with hardly any discomfort.

This was not a miracle. I'm not trying to create an "I'm healed" or "I'm amazing" story. It is simply biology and the power of the brain.

Remember when I said the brain weighed imminent tiger attack versus sprained ankle and determined the tiger was more dangerous so the ankle pain signal was not given? My brain weighed child in life-or-death situation versus pain from c-section and decided that my child's emergency was more important and that my abdominal pain could be felt later (and YES, let me reassure you that the pain did return, almost immediately when I got upstairs and saw that the twins were stable).

Does this happen to every mom? No. And more importantly, does that mean if you couldn't get to the NICU because your pain was too much that your brain did not feel your baby was more important? *Emphatically, NO, it does not mean that.* I could go on to tell you story after story of patients I've treated who could not get to the NICU until their pain was more under control, and these women are amazing mothers for whom I have the utmost respect. It's just MY story to illustrate how powerful the brain is so that we can recognize the importance of addressing it during your baby's NICU stay.

So, let's go back to the tiger. If you haven't already figured it out, the NICU and all of its stresses and emergencies are the tiger. Every time an alarm sounds: tiger. Bad news from the doctor? Tiger. Thought you were going home, but something has changed and you are now staying a few more days? Another tiger.

The problem is, our body's "fight, flight, or freeze" system is designed for short bursts of time such as during an emergency. Thinking back to my NICU stay, I was in this mode for 122 days (and then more, after we went home). You do not want your brain and your hormones to be fighting and running every minute of every day during your baby's NICU journey. Why not? Think back to how your body responds. Elevated heart rate and blood pressure for days, weeks, months. Inability to focus, feeling on edge, difficulty with learning and memory. GI dysfunction like constipation or diarrhea because your body does not consider your GI function all that important when racing from the raging beast of the NICU. Difficulty sleeping (not important when running away). Lowered immunity (this can be a big one because while your body thinks it's not important to be safe from infections during an emergency, all NICU mamas know this is THE most important thing with a baby in the NICU).

Yes, there are going to be many bursts of sprinting from a tiger in the NICU; it goes with the territory. What we want to try to improve, though, is continually running with no breaks for your entire stay.

Quick side note: If your NICU baby is now older and you've been home for a while, please don't disregard this chapter. My kids are eight, and I still catch myself constantly worrying. You can use these techniques at any time in your life to address whatever your life's "tiger" is during that time. It may not even be your kids. It could be work or finances. These tips will help you take control over anything that is keeping you in "fight, flight, or freeze."

So, what can you do? Follow the tips below to begin the journey of calming your mind and its physiological responses. If high levels of anxiety remain, please mention this to your doctor or find a local mental health professional to provide you with an individualized treatment program.

1. **Diaphragmatic breathing (yep, again):** Breathing is awesome because it is the one part of this system that we can actually control. We can't tell our heart to stop racing or our palms to stop sweating, but we can control our breathing and when our breathing slows, the other physiological responses will follow. I suggest learning this technique while laying down, but NICU mama, it can easily be done sitting or standing by your baby's isolette. You may have already begun this exercise to address something else earlier in the book. Now, it has another purpose! Inhale through your nose for two seconds and focus on expanding the abdomen and raising the ribs up and out. Then, exhale through your mouth as if you are gently blowing out birthday candles for two to four seconds, letting your belly and ribs come back down. When patients ask how much to do this, I tell them you can't do it too much. Create time to do 5-10 minute sessions a couple times a day and then add in additional

use of it whenever you start to feel your stress level rising. Here's my favorite part of this technique! If you are in a position in the NICU where you are allowed to hold your baby, do this then. This is especially important for our tiniest preemies who are on oxygen support. Even if they are on ventilators, holding them skin-to-skin and performing slow, deep breathing has been shown to stabilize babies' respiratory and cardiac systems. Treatment for mom and baby at the same time!

2. **Mindfulness:** We live in a hurried society where a fast-moving pace and increased productivity are placed on the highest pedestal. Most of us, myself included, have spent years working our tails off in school or the workplace to earn what we want and often, taking time to slow down is just not figured into the schedule. I don't sit still well. Even if I am sitting still, I'm reading or writing or completing some other task that just needs doing. It often takes my husband directly confronting me and telling me to unplug and just sit and watch a movie with him. So, I'm a work in progress, but I have learned the benefit of mindfulness while working with patients suffering from chronic pain. It's now a technique I use myself, and I *really* wish it was one I had been taught while the twins were in the NICU (and even after coming home).

   Mindfulness is basically stopping to be in the moment. It's that simple. It's slowing your mind from thinking about the next thing you're going to do or worrying about the future. Mindfulness is being present in your world at *that exact moment.* My favorite technique is to use your five senses.

   1. Stop and perform a few diaphragmatic breaths.
   2. What do you see in the moment? If you're on a walk outside, maybe you notice a tree that's leaves are beginning to change color. Maybe you notice a neighbor's dog in the window or

an especially vibrant sunset. Let's think NICU. There a lot of tubes, wires, and machines, and if you choose to notice these and it does not trigger you, then that's fine. You can also look closer, however. Look at your baby. Just look. Don't worry, don't ask questions, just look. Look at your little one's tiny fingernails. A wrinkle in his skin you may not have noticed before. Clear your mind of everything else and just look.

3. What do you hear? It's the NICU, so let's face it, we all hear the beeps. I challenge you to try to hear beyond that (this is best done when your baby is stabilized; stick with diaphragmatic breathing if your baby is having a tough moment). Can you hear an older baby cry down the hall? Do you hear a nurse laugh? Do you hear the air conditioning kick on or the roll of a cart? Do you hear someone pumping?
4. What do you smell? Is it the antiseptic that the hospital uses? Could it be a bit of the hand cream you used this morning? Is it the soap and sanitizer you used while scrubbing in?
5. What do you feel? Bonus if you are able to touch your baby in this moment, but it's still very doable if you can't! Can you feel the softness of your flannel shirt? The rubbery touch of the recliner? What do you feel if you touch your baby or if you can't touch, what if you touch the outside of the isolette?
6. What do you taste? This can be a bit more difficult at times, but maybe there's a hint of your toothpaste or something you ate for lunch. This might be better done during your small

breaks when you eat your snacks or when you go home to dinner at night. Slow down and really taste your food. It will aid with digestion and help calm the entire nervous system.

7. I like to end with a couple more deep breaths and saying something kind to yourself. It can be a mantra such as "I am strong" or "one minute at a time." It can be something kind such as "you are a good mom" or "you're doing your best in a really super tough situation." Sometimes, it's hard for us to speak kindly to ourselves, but I want you to speak with the same love that you would use to speak to your new baby.

3. **Progressive relaxation:** Began by laying down in a comfortable position (or again, you can make it work sitting in a NICU recliner). Start with a few slow, deep breaths. Then, begin to address each part of your body from the top of your head down to the tips of your toes. Start by scrunching your eyes together for five seconds. Then, unscrunch your eyes and focus on relaxing this area. Repeat by scrunching up your nose for five seconds, then let go and focus on relaxing. Move slowly one area at a time down to your toes by contracting and relaxing your shoulders, then your arms, hands, abdomen, glutes, thighs, and feet.

[illegible] when you [illegible] Slow [illegible] your [illegible] with [illegible]

7. [illegible]

3. **Progressive relaxation:** [illegible] muscle [illegible] your [illegible] area [illegible] your eyes [illegible] and [illegible] your nose [illegible] and focus on relaxing. Move slowly [illegible] area [illegible] by contracting and relaxing your shoulders [illegible] as [illegible] and [illegible]

Questions

1. Stop and assess how you feel in this moment. Is your breathing fast or slow? Is your heart racing? Do any muscles feel clenched?

2. How have you been sleeping?

3. Do you feel clear-headed? Have you had difficulty remembering things or understanding new information?

4. How has your digestion been?

5. Try mindfulness by focusing on your five senses. Assess how you feel before and how you feel afterward.

Chapter 5:
Coping with ALL the Emotions

Some of us have more warning than others, but no one, when they realize they are pregnant, plans on their baby being in the NICU. The age-old description of the NICU journey is that of a roller coaster, which I can go along with. I would also call it turbulence since often, you don't get the preparation before the sudden drop that you get with a roller coaster; you just instantly feel yourself plummet and experience that horrible heart-jumping-up-into-your-throat feeling. However you choose to describe it, we all know you need to hang on to something because it's going to be a new and frightening ride.

Fear. Guilt. Helplessness. Anger. Sadness. Loss.

It is completely okay to feel any or all of these things. You may feel one emotion one minute and another the next and that is *normal.* This is the first very important thing to realize. Your new baby is in a box, attached to tubes and wires, and you do not have to pretend that everything is okay. You have permission to really feel these feelings and know you do not have to "be positive" and "put on a happy face" all of the time. That being said, you need to feel these emotions, *but* you also need to address these emotions so that you can best care for yourself and your baby.

Side note here: I am a pelvic floor physical therapist, NOT a mental health professional. These are suggestions to try that have worked for myself and patients in similar situations however if you are struggling with anxiety, depression, OCD, or any feelings you notice that are becoming overwhelming, please reach out to a qualified professional for help. NICUs often have social workers and chaplains on staff who are more than willing to either help you themselves or refer you to another practitioner.

Ideas to try...

1. **The Ten-Minute Timed Release:** This is a technique that I also use for my patients who suffer from chronic pain or are balancing other major stressors in their lives. It is a technique I wish I had learned before my journey in the NICU, but I want to share it with you now in hopes that it might help someone else. Set a timer for 10 minutes to honor the emotions you are feeling without any judgement or filtering. Some people like to write with pen and paper, others like to type on their laptop, and others prefer to just talk out loud. Do whatever works best for you. During those ten minutes, let it all go. Write about every fear, every injustice, the anger your feel when you hear someone complain about their aches and pains at the end of their pregnancy, how you want to scream at Aunt Karen that it's *not* okay to say "at least you have a free baby-sitter for a while." Free write, free talk, punch a pillow, whatever you need to do in that moment. Don't edit your thoughts and throw grammar out the window. The purpose is not to create a beautiful essay, it's to acknowledge your emotions and let them out so that they do not stay bottled up inside your body. When the timer goes off, stop, lay down if possible and breathe. Your breaths may be shorter and shallower after moving through such intense emotions, but focus on slowing and deepening your breathing. Close your eyes and think of one thing you are thankful for in that moment. It can be something big, like the support of your sister, or something small, like the nice man who held the door open for you today when you were carrying your bags into the hospital. Just think of a little something so that by the end of the exercise, you feel a bit more at peace with just a glimmer of gratitude or hope. How many times you do this exercise each day is up to each person and where they are in their journey. When I think back to our early days in the NICU, I feel like twice a day might have been a good number for me, maybe moving down to once a day toward the last couple months of our stay when the kids were more stable, but that is not a prescription

for everyone. Do what you feel you need, and it may be different each day, and that is okay. Acknowledge that you are traversing something incredibly challenging, and you do not have any responsibility to hide your emotions to make someone else feel more comfortable. Oh, and if your NICU journey is years in the past? Use this technique when you can't handle your boss at work. Use it when your kids have used up every last ounce of patience you have. This is one of my favorite techniques to counteract the stress and strong emotions that will be inevitably present in life.

2. **Stop and check in with your body:** Often, when we are under tremendous amounts of stress, physiological symptoms begin to manifest because of either tense muscles or a more alert nervous system. Never mind the fact that you may have been on bedrest for a week (or eight) and now spend each minute standing or sitting next to an isolette. Stop and just check in with your body, head to toe. Are your shoulders clenched up toward your ears? Take a deep breath and let them fall back down. Are you thirsty? Hungry? Time to take a break in the parent room to replenish. Does your back ache from all of the standing and sitting? Try some gentle stretches. Can't quiet your mind? Try the mindfulness exercise. Are you feeling really and truly physically, mentally, and emotionally exhausted? It's okay to go out of the hospital and take a walk. I never allowed myself to do this, but mamas, *it is okay.* Does going outside seem too far away (or too cold if it's winter)? Walk down to the hospital lobby, go grab a yogurt in the cafeteria, step out and call your best friend. You'll come back feeling more centered and will be better able to focus and care for your baby.

3. **Be, don't do:** I'll be honest, I struggled with this in the NICU and I struggle with it to this day. What I mean by be, don't do is that we don't always have to be doing something. Sometimes, we

should just sit and be still. Sit and watch your baby breathe. Sit and look outside the window of the NICU. Every moment does not have to be productive. Again, I am a work in progress here. I am literally typing this chapter from a balcony overlooking the beach while on a vacation with my husband (yes, mamas, at some point, you can have a kid-free vacation again) because I do not unplug well. My husband is sleeping, and I am up early because I can't wait to put words to paper, but like I said, work in progress. You don't have to be googling and reading your preemie book every minute while you are in the NICU to gain further information. By all means, do read the book and learn what you need to know, but you can also pause. It's okay if you aren't learning abbreviations every minute (PDA, CPAP, IVH, etc.) You will learn what you need to in time, but take time to pause and just sit in the moment. Let your brain come a bit down out of it's frantic "I have to learn everything about a baby in the NICU in five days" state (I may have pictured myself eight years ago when I coined that phrase). Your baby will be just as loved and cared for if you pop in your headphones to mellow out a bit. Your balance may be different than your NICU neighbor's. Totally fine. Different baby. Different mama. Find you.

4. **Find your NICU tribe:** This is so important and can be bit tricky, but I have some tips. First of all, if you find someone who has been through a similar journey AND you feel that their personality/attitude is one which will help you, this can be amazing. When we had our twins at 24 weeks, I had two acquaintances who stepped forward to share their stories. One was the wife of one my husband's coworkers and one was a friend of a friend. While both I've learned are wonderful women, I didn't really have much contact with them prior to our delivery. When they heard about our situation, though, they came forward to talk about their similar stories and presented themselves as open to talk or answer questions.

Please note how very different this is than when others (often, people you don't even know) give advice when in fact, they have not experienced the NICU themselves. Many are well-intentioned, but you just have to deal with it however you feel in the moment and never feel like you have to tell your story when you don't want to or say/do anything to make someone else feel more comfortable. Our twins were born in June and our friends held a baby shower for us in September, when they had been in the NICU for three months. We finally had to finish our registry at one of the big block baby stores. The twins had been due in October, and our paperwork that went with the scanner said "Baby twins due October 6th." When I went in to scan in September, I was obviously not 36 weeks pregnant with twins. At the first store, the employee seemed a little confused, but she was kind and didn't say anything so I ended up telling her an abbreviated version of our story and it was all a very positive experience. At the second store, the lady gave me a snarky look like I was going to steal her scanner because obviously, I must be lying about the twins or their due date or something so I just walked away. I didn't feel like I had any responsibility to tell her our story, and it wasn't worth my time or emotions. You have full permission to walk away, ladies, this is *your* journey, and you have to protect yourself. This is your chance to allow Mama Bear to come out because even if your little one is still in the hospital, you are still a mom and protecting your child and your family is what you will do from now until forever. Use the Internet, but use it very, very carefully. As with everything online, there are incredible resources and communities for NICU mamas out there and there are some where people just go when they are frustrated or sad. When I had the twins, I immediately joined two micropreemie groups on social media, but after a couple weeks, I realized that I wasn't ready for that. I was overwhelmed. Not every baby has every issue, and I felt like I was having it all thrown at me. I left those groups for probably a couple years and have now joined them again, more to give advice when new NICU mamas ask questions. Also, since our journey, there have been some incredible women who have created some very helpful platforms that I am happy to vouch for, and I have included these in the Resources section. A good online community should make you feel supported and give you hope. There should be strict regulations controlled by an administrator so there should not be any judgement, bashing, retaliation, or attempts to sell products. If it doesn't feel right, high tail it out of there. You have no obligation to be part of any group. Be particular about your tribe and who you let influence your thoughts and your day because you, mama, are worth it.

5. **Gratitude journal:** The idea of a gratitude journal, especially if you are in the middle of a particularly stressful time in your life, may make you roll your eyes, but bear with me because I promise you it works. This has helped my patients who are overwhelmed new mamas (even without NICU stays) and patients with chronic pain. One way to keep a gratitude journal is to list three things each morning that you are thankful for. It can be something big such as "I'm thankful for my partner," but I encourage you to find smaller details. For example, maybe you write "when my partner turned the shower water on for me so it was hot when I got in." You can be thankful for big things in the NICU, like your baby coming off bilirubin lights or something small like when the unit secretary gave you an especially nice smile when you arrived. Another way to use a gratitude journal is at the end of the day which is my personal favorite because I feel it helps in two ways. First of all, I think it is a beautiful end to the day to think back through everything that happened and make note of the things that made me feel good. Secondly, when I got in the habit of writing down what I was thankful for at the end of the day, I caught myself noticing these moments

more when they occurred. Something might happen during the day, and I would think, "I'll have to write this in my gratitude journal tonight," which helped me appreciate it in the moment. Now, this is a book for NICU mamas, so let's face it, some days are disasters and it can be hard to even find three things that were good. If this is you on any given day, grab your phone and flip back through your photos. Find three happy memories that you are thankful for. Maybe it's the trip you took last year, maybe it's your pet, maybe it's a loved one you haven't seen in a while. Focus on how those moments or people made you feel, and write those memories down in your journal.

6. **Self-care:** Don't stop reading! I think if someone had mentioned self-care to me when my twins were in the NICU, I would have turned and walked away or thrown something at them, depending on my mood. Remember, though, self-care does not have to be long, luxurious, or expensive. If you can afford a one-hour massage and are open to carving out that time, that is wonderful and by all means, I completely encourage you to do that. However, if you were like me, and that wasn't going to happen, don't think self-care is not an option. Taking a shower can be self-care. Buying your favorite hand lotion because the scent makes you happy is self-care. Taking an extra 20 seconds to warm up the water before you wash your face can be self-care (I use this one a lot). There is no set amount of time or money that is required for something to be considered self-care; instead, it's anything that gives you just a little spark of joy or rest. Have 30 minutes? Go for a walk. Journal. Take a nap. Cook (if you enjoy it). Use a face mask. Listen to a podcast. Have 3 minutes? Do one yoga stretch. Pet your dog. Wear your favorite socks. Jam out to your favorite song. Whatever you can do, whenever you can do it, take the time for yourself and, indirectly, for your baby.

7. **Follow-up with your physician:** During our NICU journey, I was able to use the resources I had to make it through, taking it day by day. By staying in movement all of the time, I realize now I never allowed myself to grieve; to grieve the rest of my pregnancy and how I thought delivery would go. I had never stopped to work through the trauma of my delivery and the months to follow. My days were so full that I was able to stay on top of things for a couple years, but once the twins were around two years old and finally more medically stable, my brain began to process all we had been through. I developed severe anxiety. I was terrified any time we went anywhere in the car because I was petrified of car accidents. I kept picturing my car crashing off the side of the road. I could manage to get the twins to doctor's appointments, however I was completely unable to take them anywhere I didn't deem necessary, such as to a store, because I was sure we would have a deadly accident going somewhere that I didn't really need to go. I had completed triathlons for years by this point and despite my love for riding my bike, I couldn't bring myself to do it because I knew I would crash or be hit by a car. I kept most of my feelings inside and on the few occasions that I did mention something, my husband (who is a wonderful, caring person!) had a hard time trying to understand. I finally began to realize this new anxiety likely stemmed from the trauma we experienced in the NICU however since it had developed a couple years later, I didn't understand how it all came together. I suffered for a couple years, forcing myself to drive even though I was terrified. After thinking, reading, and researching, I began to understand how trauma is often processed after the fact, once the brain feels safe enough to really think through everything that happened. I finally gathered the courage to bring it up at my annual appointment with my primary care doctor. I explained what had happened with the twins and what I was experiencing years later. He prescribed a low-dose anti-anxiety medication

that I eventually increased in dosage until we reached the right amount. I continue to work through my anxiety with writing, reading, mindfulness, and yoga, but I also continue to take my daily anti-anxiety medication to help me cope with everything that happened, and I am not the least bit ashamed of this. Medication is not right for everyone and there are many other types of treatment, such as talk therapy, and what is right for one person may not be right for the woman sitting near the isolette next door. I do, however, hope to help squash the stigma associated with medication needed for mental health disorders. In my particular case, medication has helped me to regain some balance so that I can enjoy each day with my twins without constantly worrying about the next potential catastrophe. I no longer avoid activities because they involve riding in a car that might crash. Having a baby in the NICU can certainly be a trauma that can lead to anxiety and PTSD. If you are struggling with your emotions, whether your baby is currently in the NICU or your little one is now ten years old, please seek help from a qualified professional such as your primary care provider. You can find additional help in the Resources section at the end of the book.

Questions

1. Try the ten-minute timed release. Did you find it difficult or easy? How do you feel afterward? Do you think this might be helpful for you?

2. Describe the top three emotions you feel on a regular basis. Does anything suggest a need to work through trauma associated with your NICU stay (or any other experience)?

3. Do you have a NICU tribe? Do you feel better or worse after spending time with them?

4. Make a list of some ways you can perform self-care. I suggest making categories, such as what can be done if you have 2 free minutes, 5 free minutes, 10 free minutes, and 30 free minutes.

5. Find a notebook and keep a gratitude journal for a week. How do you feel? Does this feel like a habit that might help if you continue it?

Chapter 16:
Returning to an Active Life

My twins were in the NICU for 122 days (about four months), and so I began to return to real life and physical activity before they came home. If your NICU stay was on the shorter side, you may start to return to activity when your baby is home. If you are a NICU long-hauler, it may happen while you are still traveling to and from the hospital. Either way, you were pregnant, you gave birth, and let's face it, life has just been turned completely upside down, even if it's in a good way.

So, here's what I did. I tell you this to basically give you a demonstration of what NOT to do. If you're already past this point and you did what I did, no worries. I just want to use my story as an example to help the new moms that are still in the trenches.

My mind was on my babies, and I was stressed (see Chapter 14, that tiger was chasing me everywhere, day and night). I was a physical therapist and should have "known better," but as we all know, throw in an emergency with your child and none of us think the way we should (and how "should" we really think when our child's life is in danger? I don't think there is a true "should"). My brain was fully immersed in all of the medical terminology I was learning, the research I was doing, the pumping, the standing vigil beside two isolettes, the balancing a little bit of work in the mornings, and my stress outlet became what it had always been – running. I don't remember when I returned to running, but it was far, far too early. If I had to guess, it was around six weeks post-partum, and again, I tell you this to encourage you NOT to do this and here is why. Whether you had a vaginal delivery or a c-section, it takes 12 weeks (or more!) for tissue to heal! That means, if you had a c-section, a vaginal tear, or an episiotomy, that tissue is not even healed yet for several months. If you had none of these, don't forget that the placenta was attached to your uterus and left behind an area the size of a small dinner plate that is also healing. In addition…your pelvic floor, mamas, your pelvic floor. After delivery, these muscles can have increased tension or incredible weakness and pushing your body to do a strenuous activity like running before your pelvic floor can properly relax and contract can set you up for a whole host of problems such as incontinence, pelvic organ prolapse, and painful intercourse. In addition, there is no way that at six weeks post-partum (with no rehab) my lower abdominals were ready to support my back and hips, and I pretty much just lucked out that I didn't end up with terrible back pain after I returned to running. I just knew that I felt like the stress was going to cause my head to explode and it was something I could do for thirty minutes that would bring my anxiety down one small notch. Nobody told me not to, including my friends in the field, because I think they were almost afraid of me and what I was going through. But mamas – I was not healed and my body was not ready for that. If you are like me and you are further down your NICU road and you did what I did, it's okay. We all handle our stress in whatever way we can, but I want to take this time to try to catch our current NICU mamas in the early stages to help them do this in a way that is kinder to their bodies.

First of all, I know it sounds so incredibly simple, but you want to begin with breathing and walking. Once you are cleared to be up and moving around your hospital room (no matter how you delivered), begin to get up and walk to and from the bathroom. From there, when you are cleared, you can take your wheelchair to the NICU and walk around your baby's NICU area. If your pain is under control and your balance is good, you can then begin walking to and from the NICU. Obviously, this is going to depend on your hospital and how far apart your room and the NICU are located. I was lucky in that I was the last room at the end of the mother/baby hall so I could walk a short distance to the elevator and take it straight up to the NICU where I could walk into the twins' room (clutching my tiny vial of hand expressed milk). Once you are released from the hospital and feel ready to start more activity, continue with walking as your form of exercise. Keep it short for the first week or so after delivery and then if it feels good, slowly increase your walking time by a couple minutes and walk twice each day.

As early as is comfortable (unless otherwise directed by your physician), I begin to instruct all of our post-partum mamas (any type of delivery at any week's gestation) to do one of my very favorite exercises, the "zip-it-up" technique. Remember to keep this muscle activation gentle and pain-free, paying extra attention if you are early in your post-partum journey.

The zip-it-up technique: If you tell someone (at any time, not just during pregnancy or post-partum) to contract their abdominals, you will often see a lot of squeezing in the middle or upper abdominals (beneath the ribs) with less engagement of the lower abdominals below the belly button. Go ahead and try this on your significant other or BFF. This becomes even more apparent in pregnancy and post-partum because, well, you just *grew a human* (nice work, mama!) and your body has been through more changes than it ever has before. Go ahead and place your hand on your lower abdominal muscles underneath your belly button. Try to give a very small squeeze. Do you feel anything? If not, don't worry, you are in the majority, and we can fix this, starting with this technique. Imagine that you have a zipper that starts around your pubic bone in the front and it zips up your lower abdomen to your belly button. Inhale using your diaphragm, expanding your rib cage and belly out. Exhale through your mouth and then contract your lower abdominal muscles gently by zipping from the pubic bone to the belly button. Remember, the upper and middle abdominals are often stronger and more easily activated so don't allow those to take over. Try putting a hand over your lower abdominals to make sure you feel a gentle contraction in this area and your other hand on your upper abdomen to make sure these muscles are not doing too much. Hold the contraction for 5 seconds and then fully relax. Begin by doing 5-10 reps of 5-second holds, 2-3 times per day in any position (such as, again, right next to the isolette). As this becomes easier, you can progress the zip-it-up technique to the following exercises. As always, clear activity with your OB-GYN however a general guideline is to progress the zip-it-up around 3-4 weeks post-vaginal delivery and 6-7 weeks post-c-section.

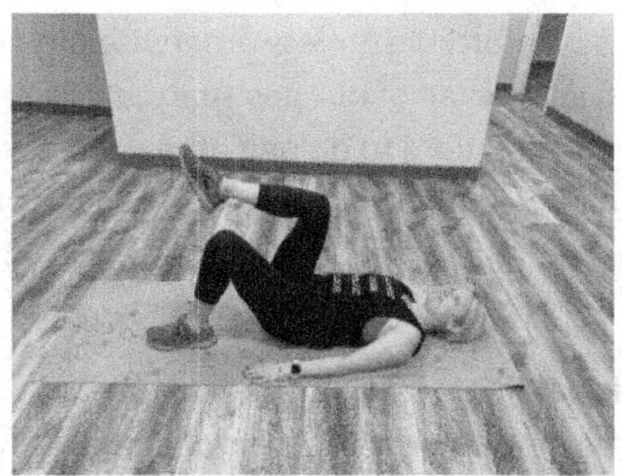

Supine marches

Supine marches: Lay on your back with your knees bent. Inhale, exhale, and zip up the lower abdominals. Raise one bent knee up to 90 degrees of hip flexion, then back down. Raise the other one up and back down. Then, relax the zipper. Continue to breathe throughout the exercise. When this becomes easy, progress the number of reps you complete while keeping the lower abdominals engaged.

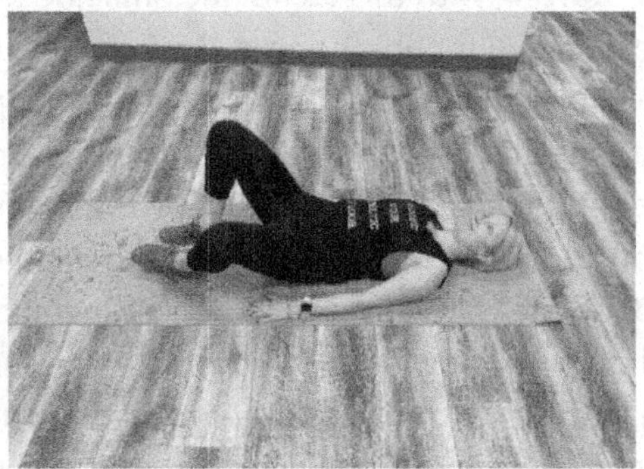

Bent knee fall-out

Bent knee fall-out: Lay on your back with your knees bent. Inhale, exhale, and zip up the lower abdominals. Let one knee fall about 45 degrees out to the side, keeping the abs engaged and not letting the hips rock. Bring the knee back up and repeat on the opposite knee (abs are still engaged, and don't forget to breathe). Relax. When this becomes easy, progress the number of reps you complete while keeping the lower abdominals engaged.

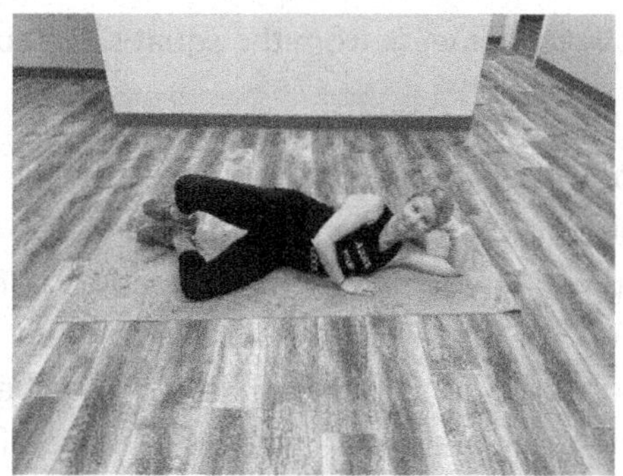

Clamshells

Clamshells: Lay on your side with your knees bent and feet together. Inhale, exhale, and zip up the lower abdominals. Keeping the abs engaged, lift your top knee up toward the ceiling and then back down. Don't let yourself roll backward! Keep the abs engaged while lifting up the top knee 5-10 times. Repeat on the opposite side. You should feel your abs engaged and your glute muscles working.

Returning to low-impact exercise: I would consider low impact exercise walking, elliptical, swimming, biking (start on a stationary bike), and lifting light weights. This does NOT include running, plyometrics, jumping jacks, or lifting heavy weights. Walking is one of the best exercises you can do as you recover. If your baby is in the NICU, find what works best with your schedule. Some mamas like to get up and go on a walk before going to the NICU. Other mamas take a break from being in the NICU and walk the hallways to help them decompress and recharge. Some mamas like to walk in the evening. There is no right or wrong time – do whatever works for you and your family. If you are feeling good a few weeks after delivery, you can begin to start some very light strength training. Remember – VERY important – to protect your healing body, always blow out when you do the hardest part of the exercise. For example, if you are doing a bicep curl, breathe in first and blow out while you curl the weights up. For a squat, the hardest part is usually standing up from the squat so be sure to blow out when you stand.

Start with body-weight resistance only, especially for lower body strengthening. Be sure to remember proper posture (ribs over pelvis – see Chapter 1) and keep your lower abdominals zipped to at least 40% with strength training and 20% for cardio like walking or riding a stationary bicycle. For long-term NICU stays, several exercises can be done right in your NICU room, and these are shown on the next several pages.

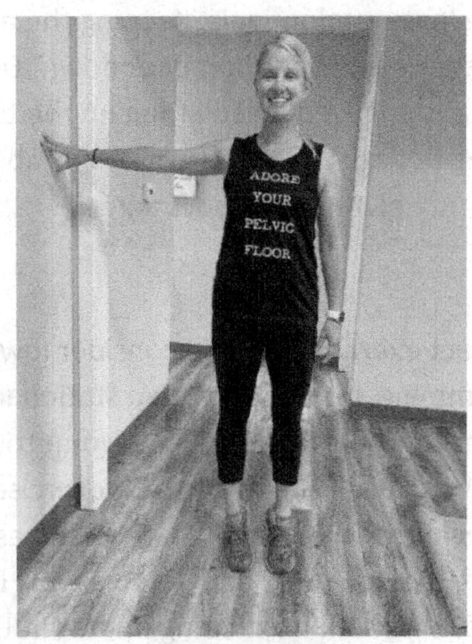

Heel raises

Heel raises: Hold on to something for support. Keeping your weight evenly distributed, raise up on to your toes and then back down. Start with 2 sets of 5 and increase over time.

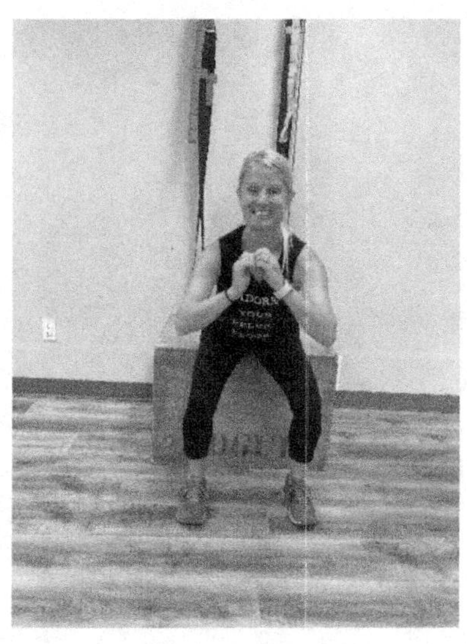

Squats to chair

Squat to chair: Keep your ribs and pelvis in line and engage your lower abdominals (zip-it-up!). Hinge your hips backward. Inhale as your lower down to touch your hips to a chair then exhale and stand back up. Keep your feet forward, your knees apart, and your tailbone back. Start with 2 sets of 5 and increase over time.

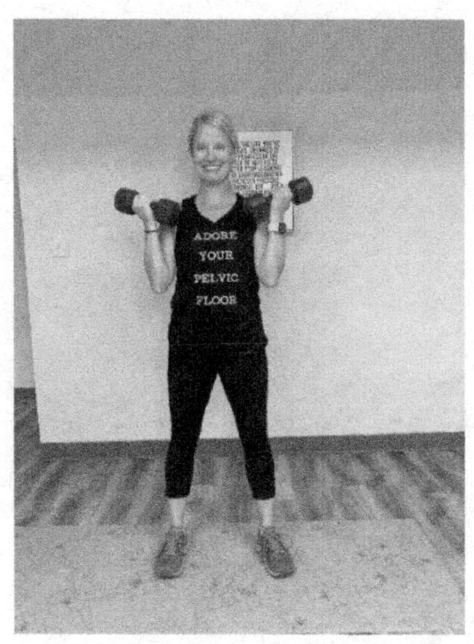

Bicep curls

Bicep curls: Stand with good posture, keeping your ribs over your pelvis and engaging your lower abs. Inhale, then exhale as you curl your arms up toward your shoulders. You can use light weights or soup cans. Inhale as you lower. Start with 2 sets of 10 and increase over time.

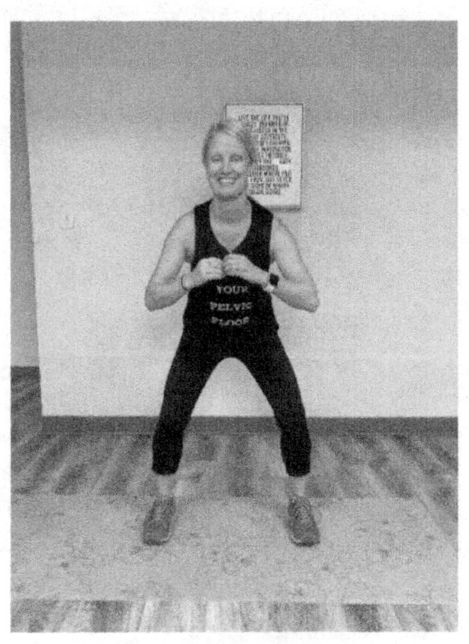

Side stepping

Side stepping: Stand in a mini squat with feet forward, knees apart, and lower abs engaged. Keep your ribs and pelvis in line, hinging your hips back. Keeping low, side step across a room one direction as far as you can and then go back the other direction.

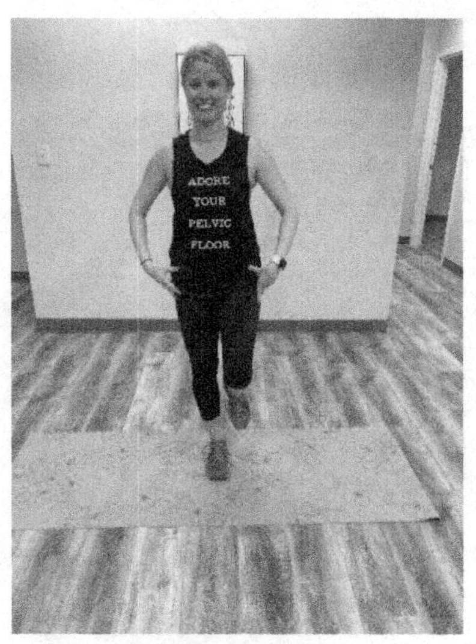

Single leg stance

Single leg stance: Keep your hips level, your lower abs engaged, and the arch of your foot lifted. Try to balance on one leg. Work up to 30 seconds on each leg.

Always stop if you feel any symptoms such as leakage, pelvic pressure, or back pain.

Returning to running/high-impact exercise: I can't tell you how many patients start to run or return to high-intensity training classes like boot camp as soon as they are released at 6 weeks. If you remember, this is what I did, too, so if you're beyond this point and you returned too early, no judgement here. However, my goal is to use this opportunity to catch new NICU mamas before they rush into things too soon, setting themselves up for future problems. Quick note! I don't want to disregard the fact that for some moms, their boot camp class or running group may be a very important social support and having a chance to go to class is helpful for their mental health. I would never want to take that away. I still encourage my patients to go to the class if this is their situation, but to complete their rehab exercises instead of high-intensity activity. It is important if they choose to do this that they feel confident they will not get caught up in the moment and do high-impact exercise before they should. My rules for mamas who want to return to running and high-intensity activities (such as jumping and plyometrics) are:

1. At least 12 weeks post-partum for full tissue healing (can be slightly variable, but this is a good general rule)
2. Can balance on each leg for 30 seconds
3. Can demonstrate good foot position
4. Can perform a series of 3 broad jumps x 3 sets without pain or symptoms
5. Has moved through glute and single-leg strengthening exercises
6. Demonstrates good pelvic floor muscle contraction and relaxation
7. Willing to complete the "Return to Run" plan, understanding the importance of stopping if symptoms occur (pelvic pressure, leakage, back pain, or anything else that does not feel right).

Let me break each of these down for you.

1. **At least 12 weeks post-partum** – pretty straight forward!
2. **Can balance on each leg for 30 seconds:** You may think this would be easy, but if it's the first time you've tried it since pregnancy, you may be surprised how challenging it can be! Test this by standing at your baby's isolette. If standing on one leg for 30 seconds is easy,

great! Move on to further steps. If it is difficult, begin by practicing standing on one leg for 10 seconds, then work up to 20, then finally to 30 seconds each. Again – all done right by your baby!

3. **Can demonstrate good foot position:** Many of us have "lazy" feet that don't maintain a good arch when we stand up. This is even more prevalent after pregnancy. Work on being aware of what your feet are doing when you sit, stand, and move. You should feel weight in the heel of your foot, on the outside of your foot, and at the base of your big toe. Try to lift your arches if you notice your feet collapsing inward toward the floor. A great exercise to do while you are sitting next to your baby in the NICU: Choose one foot to start. Try to lift just the big toe and not the four little toes. Do this 10 times. Then, try to put the big toe down and lift up just the four little toes. Do this 10 times. This will build up your foot muscles to help maintain a good arch which will then lead to good position at the ankle, knee, and hip.
4. **3 broad jumps:** Start standing (in good shoes and a good sports bra) with your feet a little wider than your hips. Bend your knees, swing your arms and jump a few feet forward, being careful to land with good knee position (don't let your knees crash in!) Your hips should be back so that when you land, your knees are not in front of you toes. Complete this series for three jumps in a row. Rest. Repeat. You should not feel any pelvic pressure or have any leakage if you are ready to return to running or high-intensity exercise.

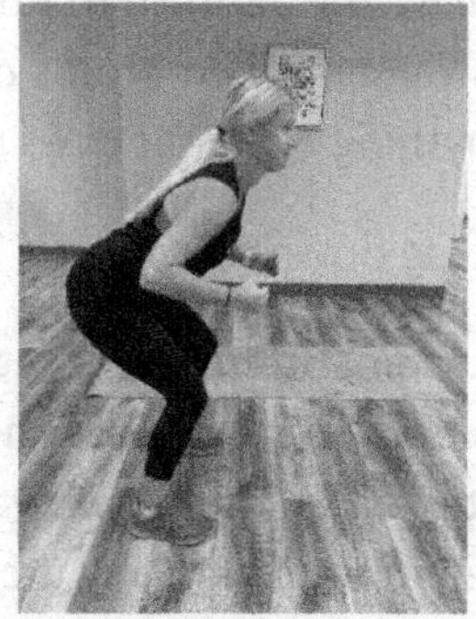

Broad jump position

5. **Glute and single-leg strengthening exercises:** Okay, I'll admit up front that many of these can't be done in the NICU like so many of our other exercises. Work into these when you feel ready and have time at home.

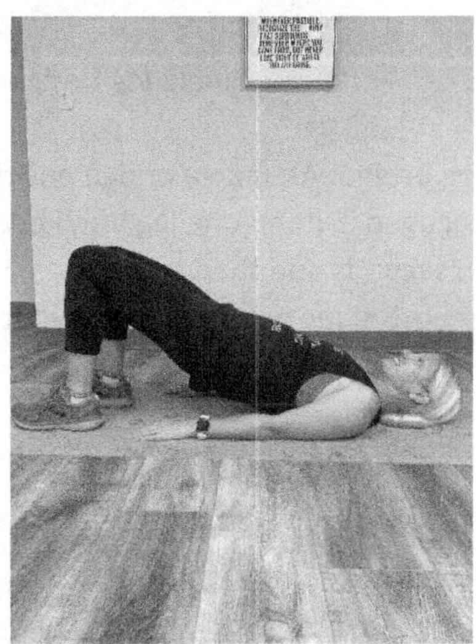

Bridge

Bridge: Lay on your back with your knees bent. Inhale, exhale and engage your lower abs and glutes. Continue to exhale as you lift your hips. Inhale again at the top keeping your muscles engaged. Exhale and lower back down. Start with 2 sets of 5 and increase over time.

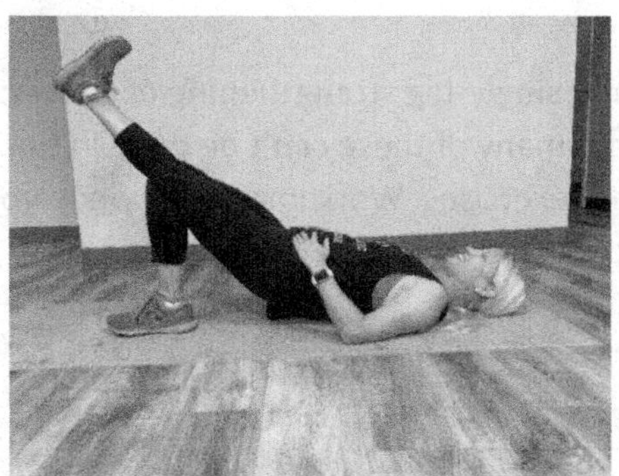

Single leg bridge

Single leg bridge: Assume a bridge position with lower abs and glutes engaged. Extend one leg out, keeping the thighs parallel. Hold for 5 seconds and then switch legs. Start with 3 reps of 5 sec holds on both sides before bringing your hips back down to the floor.

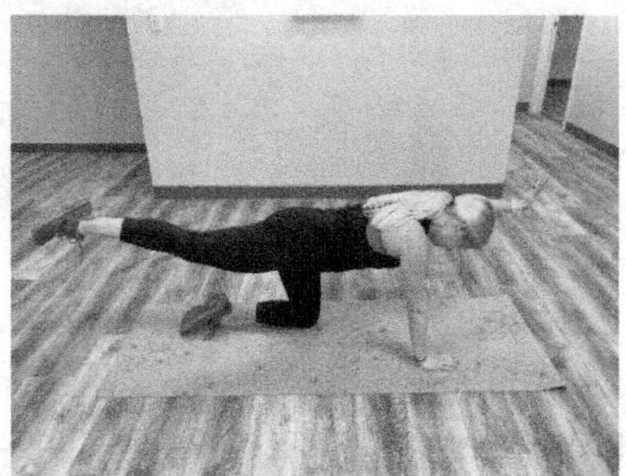

Bird dog

Bird dog: Start on hands and knees keeping your back flat and your abs engaged. Inhale, exhale and extend your left arm and right leg. Inhale and return to start. Exhale and repeat on the opposite side. Start with 3-5 reps keeping strong and stable.

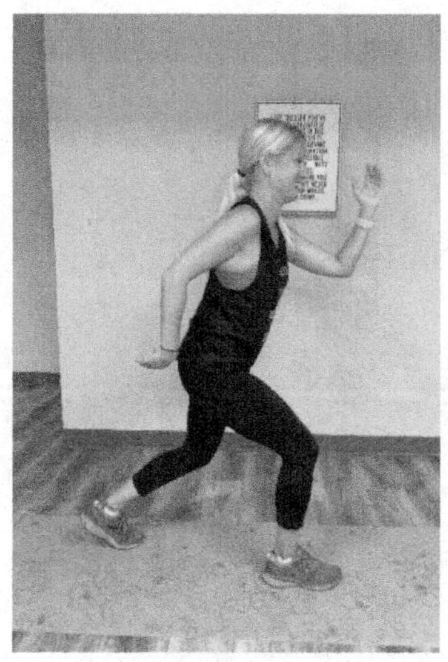
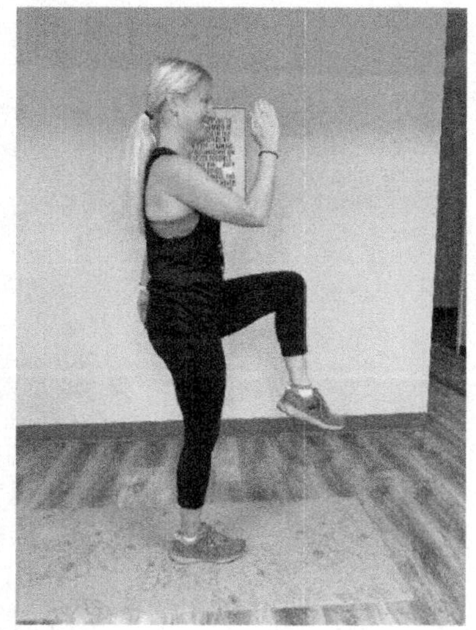

Running Man

Running man: Begin as pictured in the first photograph. Keep your lower abs engaged. Inhale and then exhale while switching your arms and bringing your back leg up into a march. You can increase the speed on this one as a progression back to running! Start with 8-10 reps on each side.

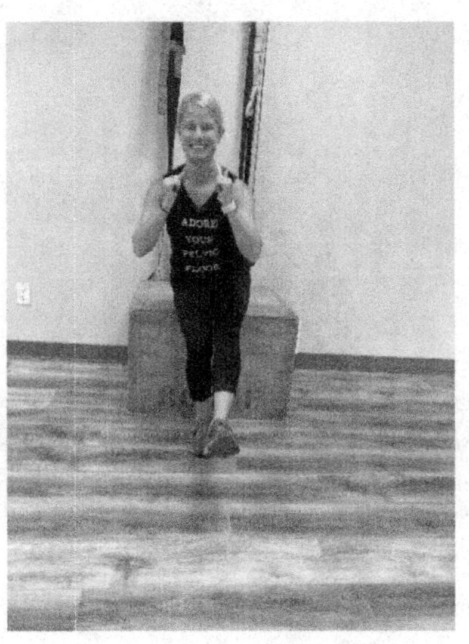

Pistol squats

Pistol squats: Stand on one leg with the other out in front. Keep hips level and lower abs engaged. Bend your knee, hinge at the hips, and sit back onto a box or chair. Without resting, use your muscles to bring yourself back up to start. Don't let your knee crash in! These are tough – start on a higher chair in the beginning and progress to a lower couch or box.

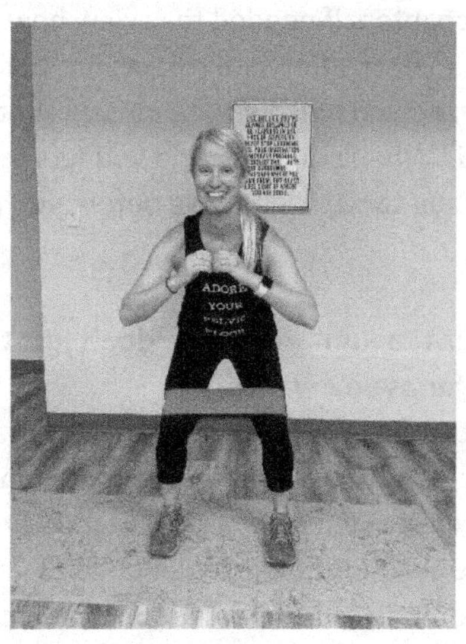

Crabwalks

Crabwalks: Stand with a resistance band above your knees. Bend your knees, keep your feet straight, and hinge at the hips to reach a mini squat. Keep your lower abs engaged as you side step all the way down a hallway or across a room. Then, come back while facing the same way (leading with the opposite leg). Repeat 2-3 times.

6. **Good pelvic floor contraction and relaxation:** Return to the previous chapters if needed to review how to properly complete pelvic floor contraction and relaxation. When you pick up a blueberry, do you feel a strong muscle contraction with a lift toward your head? When you let go, do you feel the muscles fully relax? If not, continue to work on these before you progress to high-level activity.

7. **The "Return to Run" plan (aka: don't just tie on your shoes and try to run as far as you want):**
    a. Start with five-minute intervals. Walk for 4 minutes, then jog at a comfortable pace for 1 minute (if you were not an experienced runner pre-pregnancy, you may begin with 20-30 seconds of jogging). Repeat if you feel comfortable, but don't do more than 4 rounds at first.
    b. Wait a couple days. The next time you run, you can either complete the 4/1 interval again if that was challenging or progress to walking for 3 minutes and jogging for 2. Do not progress to the next level if you are still feeling challenged by the level you are currently practicing.
    c. When ready, progress to walking for 2 minutes and jogging for 3. Later, walk for 1 minute and jog for 4.
    d. Once you can complete walk 1 min/jog 4 min for *four rounds*, you can then advance to continuous running, progressing on your own, but still being cautious to avoid doing too much too soon (too fast, too many hills, and remember – distance should increase by no more than 10% a week).
    e. The most important part? STOP IF YOU HAVE SYMPTOMS!
8. If you are returning to any other type of impact exercise (HIIT, boot camp, plyometrics), follow the same plan except you do not need to complete #7 unless you are also running.

Other considerations: Invest in a very supportive sports bra as your chest may be a larger size than what you wore pre-pregnancy, and good support is essential. Nursing sports bras are available and may be a good option. Also, make sure you are returning to high-level exercise in good, supportive athletic shoes, and these may need to be new ones since many women's feet change size and shape during pregnancy.

Advice from the NICU Mama Sisterhood

We all have such different journeys. I have been blessed to meet some incredible people including individuals on our medical teams over the years and – where I want to bring you now – other NICU mamas. I wanted to leave a section in this book for advice from one NICU mama to another. Please know that while the road is long and arduous, you are not alone and there is a sisterhood of other NICU mamas out there who welcome you with open arms.

- Have a communications team. Figure out a way to share the information you want to share and make it so you only have to do it once as opposed to answering every call, email, and text you receive. Set up an Instagram account, send a weekly email, or designate a specific person to be in charge of spreading any news you would like to share. – NICU mama

- I would say that as hard as it is to go home, sleeping in your own bed and getting rest and not pushing yourself too hard in the immediate post-partum period will allow you to be more clear-minded when you are there and to focus on the things you need to. It also helps with your milk production and hopefully avoiding complications from doing too much too fast. I call the nurse for an update right before bed, with my pumping, and in the morning which helps me sleep better knowing he is okay. – NICU mama and NICU nurse

- The most therapeutic thing is a good night's rest in their own bed and showering in their own shower. Small step, but so very important. – NICU nurse

- Learn from the nurses as much as you can. Also, remember you are still the parent and the best advocate for your child. – NICU mama

- Don't be afraid to ask a lot of questions. Take notes and write information down because it can be a lot of information at once. There were concerns that I had some issues that were related to our son's premature birth, and after he was born, I had a lot of anxiety about my health and if I was okay (adding to the stress and worry of a baby in the NICU). I made sure to contact my OB and get in for an appointment to calm my worries. When it comes to how much time you spend in the NICU with your baby, do what works best for you, your mental health, and your family. If you need to spend time at home, then do (you can always call and get updates from your nurse). If you want to be there all day, then do. My husband and I decided to have a date night before our son came home because we knew it was going to be overwhelming and stressful bringing him home on oxygen and monitors and most likely we wouldn't feel comfortable leaving him for a while. – NICU mama

- I felt that there was a lot of pressure about milk production, especially to help preemies with immunity. I ended up doing fine in the end but it was really hard on several moms. It's okay if it doesn't work for you. You are not a bad mom if you can't get the breast milk thing down. The hardest part for me was waiting to go through the feeding protocol. We could give him medication or add oxygen or do any number of things to fix different issues. But we couldn't make him eat. That had to be something he could do in his own time which was really hard for me. I wasn't good about things that I could not control. So, I want moms to know that there are some things you just can't fix which is the hardest part as a parent. But they will come along when they are ready so just take a breath. Not all forms of support may be helpful to you. And that's OK. Find someone that might be the best fit for you to vent to. For me, it was my son's NICU neighbor's parents. Our sons were medically having different issues, but probably on the same severity level, so it was a great relationship for us to foster. I am still connected to that family today, mainly on our boys' birthdays. – NICU mama

- Take it easy on yourself. Mom guilt and fear are strong, very strong even, but you are stronger. Whether it seems like it or not, you have what it takes to handle what you are facing. The NICU journey you are embarking on will really take it out of you, so take great care of yourself. It's ok to rest, eat a healthy hot meal, drink plenty of fluids, and sleep in your own bed. It will be hard at first to make yourself do these things and step away for a moment from your precious one, but it's so important because you gather strength from these basic things, as well as from your support system, the staff, and your miracle baby you would do anything for. There will be times when you feel frustrated, angry, confused, and heartbroken. First, don't forget to celebrate both the special milestones and the calm moments between those milestones. Remind yourself how this tiny person keeps overcoming the most daunting obstacles; that will help you through the setbacks and the really tough days. The staff in the NICU from the secretary who greets you, to the bedside nurse, various therapists, social workers, NNPs, and physicians all want the very best for your baby. There may be times when you feel frustrated with progress, plans, or experiences. When that happens, trust that we as a team will never rest at committing all our knowledge and experience to provide the care that will help your child reach their highest potential. Communication and trust are key, even if that doesn't come easy. – NICU mama and NICU neonatal nurse practitioner

- You have to take it one day at a time or you'll go crazy. Let your baby be the one to tell you what they are capable of. Everyone tells you to take care of yourself and they're right; it's just hard to do sometimes. Do what you can, and don't be too hard on yourself. Give grace to everyone: to the nurses, the doctors, the custodians, the secretary, your partner, your kids, and most importantly, to yourself. – NICU mama

Resources

Information about our clinic:

Empower Your Pelvis

672 SE Bayberry Lane Suite 101

Lee's Summit, MO 64063

www.empoweryourpelvis.com

In-person and virtual appointments available as well as online programs

Instagram:

@heatherevansdpt for my pelvic health account

@learningtobreathebook for my family/NICU journey

Lubricants:

Coconut oil (be aware that coconut oil can break down condoms)

Coconu (water-based, oil-based, and hemp infused)

Slippery Stuff

Good Clean Love

Pregnancy and post-partum support garments:

Bao Bei Maternity: www.baobeibody.com

Belly Bandit: www.bellybandit.com

V2 Supporter for perineal support (prolapse and varicosities)

Serola SI belts for hip and pubic symphysis pain: www.serola.net

Pelvic wands and dilators:

www.intimaterose.com, use code HEATHER12 for $5 off!

Podcasts:

Dear NICU Mama

Parenting Mighty Littles

NICU Stories

Story Sanctuary

Knock on Parenthood

Empower Your Pelvis Podcast

Squatty Potty:

www.squattypotty.com

Books:

Learning to Breathe by Heather Evans - that's me! (NICU specific)

The Preemie Primer by Jennifer Gunter (NICU specific)

Preemies – Second Edition: The Essential Guide for Parents of Premature Babies by Mia Wechsler Doron, Emma Trenti Paroli, and Dana Wechsler Linden (NICU specific)

Pregnancy Brain by Parijat Desphande (NICU and high-risk pregnancy)

The Vagina Bible by Jennifer Gunter (women's health)

Pelvic Pain Explained by Stephanie Prendergast and Elizabeth Rummer (Pelvic pain)

The Stress-Proof Brain by Melanie Greenberg (pelvic pain and stress)

What No One Tells You: A Guide to Your Emotions from Pregnancy to Motherhood by Alexandra Sacks and Catherine Birndorf (post-partum and motherhood)

The Gift of a Happy Mother by Rebecca Evans (motherhood)

Dietician resources:

Instagram @prenatalnutritionist

Instagram @nutrition_with_michal

Lactation support:

www.nurturelactationkc.com, Sarah Brock IBCLC

www.kellymom.com

Mental health support:

Post-partum Support International www.postpartum.net

To reach a suicide crisis counselor for immediate help, text 741741 or call 1-800-273-8255 (TALK)

Dr. Ashurina Ream at www.psychedmommy.com

Apps:

Mindful Mamas (mindfulness for mothers)

Calm (guided meditation)

Headspace (guided meditation)

Insight timer (guided meditation)

Down Dog (yoga)

How to find a pelvic health PT:

www.pelvicguru.com, click on Directory

www.pelvicrehab.com, click on Find a Practitioner

NICU resources:

March of Dimes: www.marchofdimes.org

Hand to Hold: www.handtohold.org

About the Author

Heather Evans is a pelvic health physical therapist, author, and mom living outside of Kansas City. She graduated from the University of Kansas with her masters of physical therapy in 2005 and doctorate of physical therapy in 2013. After a few years working in outpatient orthopedics, she has specialized in pelvic health for the past thirteen years. She currently works at Empower Your Pelvis, located in a suburb of Kansas City.

Heather became especially interested in helping post-partum mothers who had babies in the NICU after delivering her twins at 24 weeks, 1 day gestation in 2013. The twins spent 122 days in the NICU, coming home one day before their 4-month birthday.

Today, Heather enjoys balancing working in pelvic health with spending time with her husband, Brian, and her 8-year-old twins, Hannah and Gavin. She also loves competing in triathlons, reading, listening to podcasts, being near the ocean, coffee, sushi, and walking her pomsky.

Heather's full NICU story can be found in her first book, Learning to Breathe.

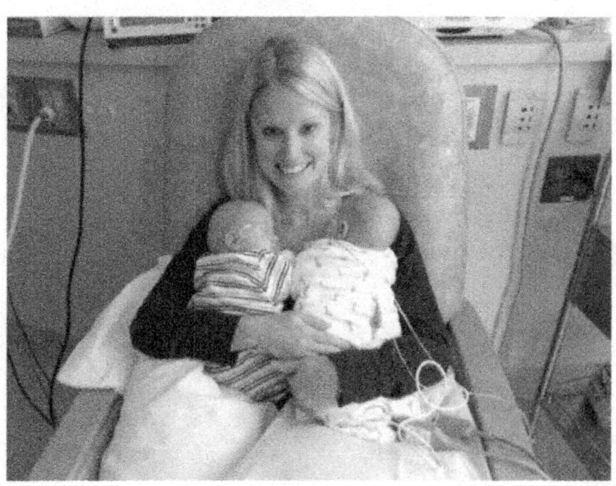

Made in the USA
Monee, IL
07 August 2025

22082523R00105